# CQI

Continuous Quality Improvement

## for

## Diabetes Education
## and Support
## Programs

## Third Edition

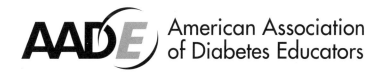

American Association
of Diabetes Educators

# Contents

*Contents*

# Acknowledgements

The American Association of Diabetes Educators (AADE) would like to acknowledge the work and contributions made to the third edition of this book by the following individuals.

## Writers

Jo-Anne Rizzotto, MEd, RD, LDN, CDE

Director, Educational Services

Joslin Diabetes Center

Boston, MA

Erin L. McGinley, BS

Research Coordinator

Penn State College of Medicine

Hershey, PA

## Reviewers

Paulina N. Duker, MPH, RN, BC-ADM, CDE

Former VP, Diabetes Education and Clinical Programs

American Diabetes Association

Laura Rooney, DNP, APRN, FNP-BC, BC-ADM, FAANP

Director, UT Health Services

University of Texas Health Science Center Houston

# Introduction

The burden of diabetes in the United States is staggering—approximately 25.8 million Americans have been diagnosed with diabetes, costing the American healthcare system approximately $245 billion.[1,2] Currently, 1 in every 5 healthcare dollars is spent on diabetes and its complications; the average person with diabetes spends $7,900 more a year on medical expenditures than a person without diabetes.[2] With the passage of the Patient Protection and Affordable Care Act of 2010 (ACA), the most significant healthcare reform since the implementation of Medicare and Medicaid in 1965 is under way. With its emphasis on improving the experience of care, improving the health of populations, and reducing the per capita costs of health care—the Triple Aim[3]—the ACA provides an opportunity for improving the delivery of diabetes care.

In a time of change, processes such as *continuous quality improvement* (CQI) help to test the change within a defined setting. As healthcare professionals strive to provide their patients with the best care possible, structured programs around CQI are critical to help raise the bar of both clinical and professional practices. This handbook is meant to provide relatable examples of how CQI can be implemented in diabetes care and education, as well as provide alternate solutions to barriers that many programs face throughout implementation.

Change is hard; improving the quality of care delivered to people with prediabetes and diabetes is even harder. Our hope is that this book can help ease the processes around implementing a CQI program that will help to better both your patients' outcomes and your own professional life.

**Note:** Traditionally, the diabetes education process has been called *diabetes self-management education or training* (DSME/T). For the purposes of this handbook, DSME will be used.

# Chapter 1 CQI and the United States Healthcare System

As professionals and organizations have attempted to define quality, many different definitions and processes to achieve it have emerged, including *quality assurance*, *quality assessment*, *total quality management*, and *process improvement* (Table 1.1).

**Table 1.1 Terms for Quality Improvement (QI)**

- Continuous improvement
- Performance improvement
- Performance management
- Process improvement
- Quality assessment
- Total quality management (TQM)
- Quality assurance
- Quality control
- Quality planning
- Re-engineering

Although there are a variety of names for and approaches to quality improvement, these programs share three common attributes:

1. Emphasis on process and systems rather than individuals
2. Recognition of both internal and external customers
3. Use of objective data to analyze and improve processes while measuring improvements

The term that will be used in this handbook is *continuous quality improvement* or *CQI*. CQI is a system that seeks to improve the provision of services with an emphasis on future results. Like total quality management, CQI uses a set of statistical tools to understand subsystems and uncover problems, but its emphasis is on maintaining quality in the future, not just controlling a process. Once a process that needs improvement is identified, a team of knowledgeable individuals is gathered to research and document each step of that process. Once specific expectations and the means to measure them have been established, implementation aims at preventing future failures and involves the setting of goals, education, and the measurement of results. If necessary, the plan may be revised on the basis of the results, so that the improvement is ongoing.[4]

Within the healthcare sector, CQI has supported improvements in the delivery of patient education, improved patient outcomes, decreased costs, and provided for more efficient care across the healthcare spectrum.[5]

Before expanding upon the shared attributes of quality improvement processes and addressing the implementation of the CQI process in your healthcare setting, a brief background on the development of quality and efficiency processes in general may be helpful.

## Evolution of the Quality Improvement Process

The scientific revolution of the 1600s is credited with the introduction and use of the scientific method (observe, hypothesize, test, analyze) in product development, while the first industrial revolution (1760–1830) is credited with the introduction and use of product standardization. By the second industrial revolution (1871–1914), application of the scientific method was a major source of improvement in every industry, as control and feedback were being used to improve the work process. Quality management evolved over this period as engineers and managers responded to work-related problems. Quality management combined the scientific method used in the field of engineering with the principles of management—control and feedback.[6]

Frederick Winslow Taylor's *The Principles of Scientific Management*, published in 1911, is recognized as the direct predecessor of quality management. The publication describes Taylor's approach to improving productivity and quality in assembly line work in factories. Taylor used engineering principles—time-and-motion studies—to select the best tools and methods for doing the job, followed by management principles to engage and train the workers to utilize these tools and methods.[6]

Walter Shewhart added statistical quality control (inspection and statistics)—now referred to as quality control (QC)—to the field of quality management. Application of statistical sampling ensured, for example, that 95%–99% of the products would meet the standards; therefore it was no longer necessary to inspect each product that came off the assembly line. Shewhart also developed the approach *Plan-Do-Check-Act* (PDCA) while working as a physicist at Bell Labs from 1924 to 1956 (Figure 1.1). The process of PDCA can be used repeatedly to improve outcomes by changing the process and improving quality. This cycle allows for quick refinement and assessment of the process, which allows for rapid improvement to continually occur throughout the cycle. The process of PDCA is sometimes referred to as the continuous improvement cycle, the Shewhart cycle, the Deming cycle, or the PDSA (Plan-Do-Study-Act) cycle.[6]

W. Edwards Deming added to the work of his colleague and protégé Walter Shewhart and pioneered total quality management (TQM), combining QC and PDSA to achieve continuous quality improvement across an entire industry rather than in one company at a time. Deming developed TQM in Japan in cooperation with Japanese scientists, engineers, and industrial leaders in large electronics and manufacturing companies beginning in the 1950s, a time when the

**Figure 1.1  Plan-Do-Check-Act (PDCA) Cycle**

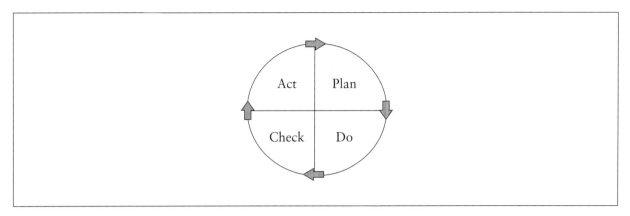

Japanese were motivated to improve economic conditions following World War II. The Japanese approach was to listen to and use the expertise of the workers, and to *fix the process, not the product*. Within five years of incorporating TQM, the Japanese were producing products that were competitive on the world market.[6,7]

Except during wartime, when there was a high demand for productivity, the United States has been very slow to adopt quality management methods. Deming suggested this reluctance to adopt quality measures stems from the following, all of which are applicable today:

1. During times of economic prosperity, business does not see a need for quality management.
2. Management-labor conflicts fueled by a culture that places a low value on the workers.
3. A focus on quick profits, whereas implementation of a quality management program requires a time investment of two to five years.[6]

By the late 1970s and early 1980s, industry in the United States had become concerned about its ability to deliver high-quality products while reducing costs in order to be competitive on the world market. The CEO of the Ford Motor Company sought assistance from Deming, who implemented quality management at Ford. This started a period of progress in quality management in North America that lasted over a decade.[7]

Other tools for quality management that have been developed over the past 20 years include ISO 9000, LEAN/Six Sigma, Gemba Kaizen for Lean or Just in Time (JIT), and other methodologies (Table 1.2). The International Organization for Standardization (ISO) is a worldwide body that sets standards for industry and certifies ISO 9000 status for a company that meets these standards. ISO is based in Europe, and its standardization process has supported the gradual economic unification of European countries. The emphasis of ISO 9000 is on product quality rather than TQM and is often required by corporate vendors as well as customers. ISO 9000 facilitated globalization of the telephone, Internet, auto, and aerospace industries.[8]

**Table 1.2  Process Tools for QI Projects**

- Plan-Do-Check-Act (PDCA); Plan-Do-Study-Act (PDSA)
- Project Definition—Diagnostic Journey—Remedial Journey—Holding the Gains
- Plan—Design—Measure—Assess—Improve
- Assess—Design—Develop—Implement—Evaluate (ADDIE)
- ISO 9000
- Six Sigma and LEAN/Six Sigma
- Gemba Kaizen for Lean or Just in Time (JIT)

Six Sigma is named after a statistical goal and is a methodology like TQM. Six Sigma engineering was developed by Motorola and General Electric, and its use is limited to the manufacturing of millions of identical products or billions of identical components, for example, in electronics or auto manufacturing, or in processing millions of checks per day in the banking industry. The sigma level refers to the number of defects per billion; for Six Sigma there are two defects per billion or 99.7% without defects.[8]

LEAN and Six Sigma are similar methodologies that seek to eliminate waste. Recently, LEAN has become adopted in the healthcare industry, with the underlying belief that waste comes from unnecessary steps in the production process.[8] Similarly, Six Sigma also looks to reduce waste, though both methodologies identify the cause of waste differently. LEAN has become popular due to the demonstrated success of the Toyota Production System.[9,10]

Quality management (QM) efforts started by Deming after World War II continue to this day, although QM has been more successful in Japan than in North America or Europe. The reason for this is that the Japanese business culture tends to focus on continuous improvement, while Western business culture tends to focus on innovation. Masaaki Imai, the founder of the Kaizen Institute in Japan, advanced TQM with Kaizen (change-good, translated as continuous improvement), Gemba (where the action is—the shop floor), and Just-in-Time (JIT) manufacturing or producing only enough to meet customer orders. In Japan, the emphasis is on improving the process, encouraging employees to suggest changes in their own work, and following PDCA to evaluate these suggestions. For example, suggested changes could be improvement in machines, tools, or processes with a savings in energy or other resources, and/or improved quality or customer services.[11]

## Quality Improvement and the United States Healthcare System

The passage of the Patient Protection and Affordable Care Act of 2010[12] (ACA) has become the most significant healthcare reform in the United States since the passage of Medicare and Medicaid in 1965. With the creation of accountable care organizations (ACOs),[13] the healthcare system seeks to tie reimbursement to outcomes and quality of care received for identified patient populations, known as population management. The overall goal of an ACO is to decrease the total costs of care delivered to the population, allowing for shared savings benefits. Another major goal of the ACO is to leverage best practices to achieve high quality across the network.

Accreditation and reimbursement are now tied to demonstrable outcome measurements and quality improvements. For example, more than 90% of US health plans use the National Committee for Quality Assurance's HEDIS (Healthcare Effectiveness Data and Information Set) tool to measure performance on important dimensions of care and quality.[14] Hospitals and other healthcare entities must address the strict quality improvement measures required for accreditation by The Joint Commission.

Nearly every part of the healthcare industry—hospitals, health plans, nursing homes, and healthcare providers like physicians, nurses, and home health providers—is sensitized to improving healthcare quality standards and reimbursement guidelines. The federal government, states, employers, labor unions, and consumer advocates are also focused on improving care. In addition, physician education and accreditation programs require training in practice improvement.[15] Required education in quality and practice improvement has added value to organizations and providers alike.[16]

As the population continues to age, there is a strong economic incentive to improve efficiency while controlling the cost of health care. The number of Americans aged 65 and older is set to double by 2030, overburdening the already underdeveloped/inadequate healthcare workforce.[17] As of 2012, almost half of the population of the United States had one or more chronic diseases, and 25% had two or more chronic conditions. Chronic conditions account for more than 80% of healthcare costs, with most of these costs being preventable.[18]

The 2001 Institute of Medicine (IOM) report, *Crossing the Quality Chasm,* identified major deficiencies in healthcare delivery, including underuse, overuse, variation in healthcare delivery, and a lack of coordinated care, especially for those with chronic diseases.[19] The IOM recommended an information technology infrastructure to support performance measurement and clinical decision making, while identifying chronic care quality improvement as a high priority.[20] In order for the United States to improve the quality of the healthcare delivery system, a collaborative national effort is needed to consolidate healthcare performance measurement and reporting, according to the IOM report.[20] Although significant gains have been made to improve the US healthcare system, there are still gaps in the system. The United States has made numerous strides, for example, in reducing bloodstream infections, but challenges still arise around adoption and implementation of best practices, along with how to measure improvement.[21]

## The Chronic Care Model

The process of changing a healthcare system from a reactive, acute care model to a proactive, Chronic Care Model (CCM)[22] relies on the effective use of CQI methods. The CCM is an evidence-based framework that delivers safe, effective, and collaborative care to patients. The organization Improving Chronic Illness Care (ICIC) has been working with national partners since the 1990s to support health systems in implementation of the CCM with the goal of improving the health of chronically ill patients.

The CCM identifies six basic areas upon which healthcare organizations need to focus to improve quality of care and delivery (Figure 1.2):

1. Health Systems
2. Delivery System Design
3. Decision Support
4. Clinical Information Systems
5. The Community
6. Self-Management Support

The system requires healthcare services that are patient-centered and coordinated among members of the healthcare staff and the patient and family. Within each of the six essential elements of the CCM, there are *change concepts* that healthcare teams can use to guide the process of changing from an acute care model to a chronic care model, resulting in improved patient and system outcomes. Characteristics of the *change concepts* for each of the six elements follow.

*Health Systems.* There is a commitment to applying the CCM across the organization beginning with the senior leaders of the organization. The organization promotes improvement strategies and open and systematic response to quality problems by including measurable goals in the strategic/business plan with aligned incentives around quality to encourage care coordination, team care, and ongoing quality improvement.

**Figure 1.2  The Chronic Care Model**

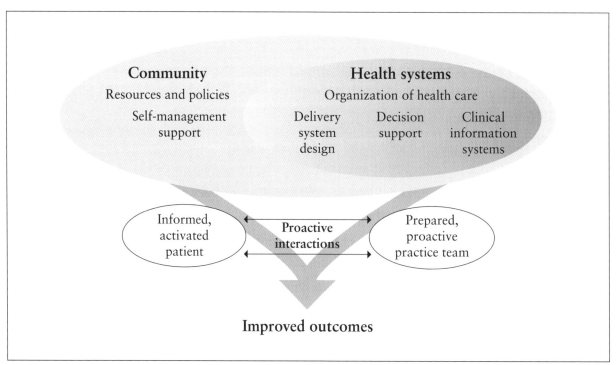

Source: Developed by The MacColl Institute, © ACP-ASIM Journals and Books, reprinted with permission from ACP-ASIM Journals and Books.

*Delivery System Design.* The organization provides effective and efficient care and self-management support with regular proactive, planned visits that utilize the skills of all care team members. This requires defining roles of team members, using evidence-based care, ensuring regular follow-up, and providing care that patients understand and is consistent with their cultural and educational background. This also includes providing patient-centered care, which encompasses interpreter services, special needs, etc.

*Decision Support.* The organization supports clinical staff in providing care based on the latest evidence-based guidelines for each chronic disease with ongoing education of clinical staff. Specialists are integrated into primary care delivery through consultation and referral networks. The staff share evidence-based guidelines with patients and encourage participation through patient activation.

*Clinical Information Systems.* The organization develops a registry of patients for each chronic disease to allow for monitoring care as well as the performance of the practice team and the healthcare system through the effective use of electronic medical records (EMRs). Outcomes are shared with both providers and patients to organize and better coordinate care while also monitoring and measuring performance outcomes.

*The Community.* Community resources, such as disease management programs, in schools, local and state governments, nonprofit organizations, and faith-based organizations are used to support patients. This also includes advocacy for policies to improve care at the community level.

*Self-Management Support.* Patients are empowered and prepared for self-management of chronic disease. Tools and resources are used to provide patients with reminders for self-management to help negotiate self-care behavior change goals through interventions with the support of peers or other professionals.

ICIC also provides the following Regional Framework to help create a "system" of better care. Below are best practices that may help increase a quality improvement program's success:

- Strong leadership committed to quality improvement
- Shared vision among clinicians and business and administration
- Routine measurement of the quality and costs of care
- Emphasis on primary care and its integration with specialty care
- Evidence-based guidelines integrated into performance measurement and clinical decision making
- Information technology that facilitates performance measurement and provides decision support for clinical care
- Organized quality improvement activities[23,24]

Research to evaluate CQI in the healthcare setting is limited, but growing. Priorities for future research include developing methods to improve patient care processes and outcomes. In 2007, the Robert Wood Johnson Foundation funded a national program (Improving the Science of Continuous Quality Improvement Program and Evaluation) to advance the science of quality improvement research and evaluation.[25] Since the 2001 IOM report, the Agency for Healthcare Research and Quality (AHRQ) has summarized results of studies evaluating quality improvement strategies for quality improvement processes involving many diseases, including diabetes.[26]

A popular care delivery model focused on providing comprehensive primary care that is closely tied to the CCM is the Patient-Centered Medical Home (PCMH). The PCMH is looked upon by health delivery systems as a CQI journey, ever changing to meet the needs of the patients. The PCMH was endorsed in 2007 by major primary care physician associations to create the Joint Principles of the PCMH.[27] Features of a medical home include patient-centeredness, comprehensiveness, and coordination and accessibility of care, as well as a commitment to quality and safety.[28] Early PCMH pilots, mostly focused around diabetes,[29] have shown improved results in patient outcomes but contradicting results in cost savings.[30,31] The movement toward PCMH practice transformation is growing as payers are beginning to enhance payments for recognized PCMH practices.[32]

## The Future of Health Care: The Triple Aim

The Centers for Medicare and Medicaid (CMS) reported slow healthcare costs for the fourth consecutive year in 2012, increasing by only 3.7% to $2.8 trillion, accounting for 17.2% of the GDP.[33] America's GDP is almost twice the average GDP on health care for the average industrialized country.[34] With the passage of the ACA, health care is focused on obtaining the Triple Aim,[35] developed by Donald Berwick and the Institute for Healthcare Improvement. The Triple Aim (Figure 1.3) was created to optimize healthcare performance at a systems level, with simultaneous pursuit of the aims to:

1. Improve the patient experience of care (quality and satisfaction)
2. Improve the health of populations
3. Reduce the per capita cost of health care

Diabetes is a critical factor as America continues to pursue the Triple Aim. Nearly 29 million people in the United States have diabetes, accounting for 8.3% of the population and 25% of senior citizens.[36] If the epidemic continues, 1 in 3 American adults will have diabetes by 2050.[37] Diabetes contributes to the healthcare cost burden as 1 in every 5 healthcare dollars is spent on

**Figure 1.3  The Triple Aim**

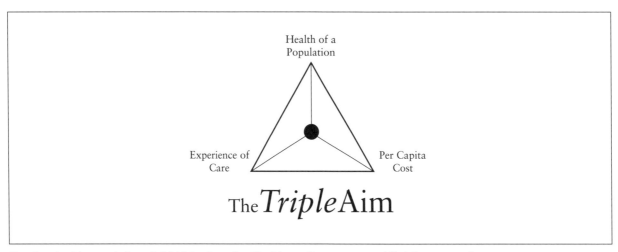

diabetes and its complications—a total of $245 billion in 2012. A person with diabetes spends $7,900 more than a person without diabetes in average medical expenditures per year.[38] The burden of diabetes continues past prevalence and costs, affecting the demand for endocrinologists. In 2010, the American Board of Internal Medicine showed that there were only 5,811 board-certified endocrinologists to serve the 6,300 hospitals in the United States.[39] As fewer physicians continue to seek endocrinology as a specialty, effective care of this growing population is threatened. Primary care also faces a shortage—an important statistic to emphasize in an aging population as over 90% of diabetes patients are treated primarily by their primary care physician.[40]

As the ACA recommends paths to success in reaching the Triple Aim, diabetes is an exemplary disease to model care after. Coordination between specialists and primary care, telemedicine to supplement the workforce, bundled payments for reimbursement models, innovative technology to manage glucose levels—all of these are examples of why the field of diabetes is both challenging and exciting to be a part of as the healthcare revolution takes shape over the next decade.

## Common Elements of CQI

As mentioned earlier in this chapter, there are three common elements shared by the various CQI processes:

1. Emphasis on Processes
2. Customer Focus
3. Use of Objective Data

### Emphasis on Processes

The focus of any CQI program is on a system's *processes* rather than the *individual*. A systems focus is one in which the analysis is on the specific processes and the relationships between those processes. The underlying assumption is that the problem is most likely caused by a system process, rather than by an individual. It is important to keep this in mind as you work through your CQI project. Evaluate the process objectively and avoid assigning blame for the problems that emerge.

### Customer Focus

Regardless of the specific CQI model used, the focus is on the customer or the user of the services. Customers may be from outside your organization or practice (external) or within it (internal). Table 1.3 shows a list of potential customers.

For many healthcare organizations, implementing effective CQI is critical for program survival. CQI efforts demonstrate commitment to quality, resource allocation, and financial viability. The universal goal of CQI is to improve health care by identifying problems and taking corrective, constructive action to overcome the problem. CQI as a management philosophy supports continually striving for excellent service and customer satisfaction in a patient-centered healthcare environment. Two underlying principles of CQI are reflected in the following questions:

1. Are consumers receiving what they want?
2. Are services being provided efficiently and effectively?

**Table 1.3  Healthcare Customers: Internal and External**

| Internal | External |
|---|---|
| Staff | Patients: outpatient, inpatient, ambulatory patients, long-term care patients, patients' families, people with diabetes/prediabetes/at risk for diabetes, healthcare consumers |
| Physicians | Providers: referring providers (physicians, nurse practitioner, physician assistant), referring specialist physicians (endocrinologists, ophthalmologists, podiatrists) |
| Directors | Payers of Care: employer groups, insurance plans, Medicare, Medicaid, occupational health groups |
| Administrators | Regulators of Care: American Association of Diabetes Educators' Diabetes Education Accreditation Program (DEAP), American Diabetes Association Education Recognition Program (ERP), Indian Health Service (IHS), The Joint Commission, Health Care Finance Administration, Centers for Medicare and Medicaid Services (CMS), Veterans Administration Health System, state health departments, Agency for Healthcare Policy and Research (AHCPR), National Committee on Quality Assurance (NCQA), Healthcare Effectiveness Data and Information Set (HEDIS) |

Identify your healthcare customers and their needs by completing the *Application to Your Practice Worksheet 1.1: Understanding Your Customers* in Appendix III.

## Use of Objective Data

A necessary element of CQI is data collection and data analysis. In all CQI efforts the data guide the decisions about programs, procedures, and future steps. Data collection can be a difficult task. Two simple questions can help guide and organize your data collection efforts:

1. What kind of data does your project want to collect?
2. How will the data be collected?

Once objective measures have been selected for monitoring, the next step is to set up a method for data collection. **Keep your data collection as simple as the needs of your project allow.** Search for tools that already exist within your institution or elsewhere before developing your own tools.

In addition, there are online resources for data collection, such as the AADE7™ Self-Care Behaviors Goal Sheet (part of the AADE7™ System[41]), the Improvement Tracker and Change Achievement Success Indicator on the Institute for Healthcare Improvement website,[42] and CQI Support Software that tracks real-time organization performance improvement by the Robert Wood Johnson Foundation[43] website.

# Chapter 2 CQI and Diabetes Self-Management Education and Support

The CQI process helps healthcare professionals achieve better outcomes by establishing or improving work processes. The Institute for Healthcare Improvement suggests three fundamental questions that should be answered by an improvement process[44]:

1. What are we trying to accomplish?
2. How will we know a change is an improvement?
3. What changes can we make that will result in an improvement?

The CQI process serves as a way for healthcare professionals to improve patient care services by examining work processes and developing closer collaboration and cooperation among interdisciplinary team members. The process benefits healthcare professionals by clarifying their specific roles and responsibilities, improving communication among the healthcare team, and establishing the framework for making and adapting to changes in the service. These beneficial and desirable outcomes of the process demonstrate the value of CQI.

In diabetes education, setting targets for educational, behavioral, and clinical outcomes is an important element of quality programs. Although behavioral and program outcomes by themselves don't constitute CQI efforts, the outcomes can be used to identify areas needing improvement in the diabetes education service and to develop worthwhile CQI projects.

Diabetes education must be responsive to advances in knowledge, treatment strategies, education strategies, and psychosocial interventions, as well as consumer trends and the changing healthcare environment. By measuring and monitoring both process and outcome data on an ongoing basis, providers of diabetes self-management education (DSME) can identify areas for improvement and make adjustments in participant engagement strategies and program offerings accordingly. Once areas for improvement are identified, the DSME provider must designate timelines and important milestones, including data collection, analysis, and presentation of results. Measuring processes and outcomes helps to ensure that change is successful without causing additional problems in the system. Outcome measures indicate the result of a process (i.e., whether changes are actually leading to improvement), while process measures provide information about what caused those results or outcomes. Process measures are often targeted to those processes that typically affect the most important outcomes.

Quality improvement is such an important process that it has been incorporated into national standards and adopted as part of certain requirements by regulatory and accrediting bodies. Diabetes education as a reimbursable service in the US healthcare system requires CQI as part of the education service. Entities seeking accreditation and reimbursement for providing diabetes education must have a quality improvement process in place to evaluate the effectiveness of the education. An ongoing CQI process is required, and evidence of the process must be demonstrated annually to the accrediting body in order to maintain accreditation or recognition and reimbursement eligibility. Currently the two national accrediting organizations are:

- Diabetes Education Accreditation Program (DEAP)—American Association of Diabetes Educators (AADE)
- Education Recognition Program (ERP)—American Diabetes Association (ADA)

Both have similar CQI requirements to attain and maintain accreditation.

The AADE and ADA have adopted the National Standards for Diabetes Management Education and Support (NSDSME/S),[45] which were developed by stakeholders in diabetes care represented by nurse educators, dietitians, primary care physicians, endocrinologists, nurse practitioners, pharmacists, people with diabetes, psychologists, and others. All AADE accredited and ADA recognized diabetes education programs are required to use a CQI process for program improvements. Evidence that an organization uses CQI can be shown in minutes from meetings or other documentation that verifies that the process and results of CQI are being implemented to improve the DSME program. Standard 10 of the NSDSME/S addresses quality improvement in DSME programs[45]:

> The provider(s) of DSME will measure the effectiveness of the education and support and look for ways to improve any identified gaps in services or service quality, using a systematic review of process and outcome data.

The CQI requirements of the American Association of Diabetes Educators Diabetes Education Accreditation Program (AADE DEAP) and the American Diabetes Association Education Recognition Program (ADA ERP) have an identified process for program performance improvement and tracking of at least 2 outcomes as a measure of program effectiveness. At a minimum, one outcome must address patient-defined goals, and the second must address any other outcomes (e.g., metabolic, clinical, quality of life, process) with a measure of attainment. Also required is documentation that results of the CQI evaluation are used to determine opportunities for improving DSME services and that a current project is in progress using that plan/process. In addition, for ADA ERP applicants (all online), a description of a formal CQI process/plan is one of 4 randomly assigned audit items that must be submitted as evidence to support application. Other audit items include:

- full copy of one assigned content area of the curriculum
- copy of one de-identified participant chart with documentation demonstrating the educational process including provider referral, assessment, education plan with goal setting, education intervention(s), evaluation of learning, follow-up with evaluation of goal achievement and

communication to referring provider including plan for diabetes self-management support (DSMS).[46,47] Competent providers need to be actively involved in the CQI process to improve a system or procedures for providing optimal care for patients.

Quality improvement techniques, or steps, are used to determine which diabetes education interventions work best to improve health, promote self-management, teach patients, and improve program outcomes. *Benchmarking*, a process of comparing current program outcomes with those of similar programs or external programs demonstrating practice standards, is a good way to measure the success of your program. Benchmarking can begin at any point that has been defined as desirable, and the outcomes can be above or below that point (Table 2.1). Having a CQI process in place contributes to improving outcomes and ensuring consistent outcomes for all patients attending the program.

Many different types of data can be collected to assess program quality. One program may measure the number of patient visits per educator, the length of visits, the most frequently selected appointment times, or the best hours for the program to operate. Another program may measure behavior change to evaluate educational impact, such as the number of times per week that participants walk more than 10,000 steps per day. The Joint Commission suggests that indicators should demonstrate effectiveness, timeliness, and efficacy. A prudent program measures indicators in each of these areas from time to time. Table 2.2 lists process measures that can be used in a CQI program. Some are examples related to patient safety required by The Joint Commission, others are required for accreditation of DSME/DSMS programs, and others are specific to a clinic or hospital.

Examining the process can identify systemic factors that either facilitate or hinder positive behavioral and clinical outcomes; for example, staff documentation is critical to monitoring achievement of positive outcomes.

## Table 2.1  Benefits of Benchmarking

1. Removing assumptions about how a process is functioning.
2. Improving understanding of competition.
3. Encouraging a search for improvement, practice breakthrough, and achievement of superior performance.
4. Revealing a more accurate picture of customer requirements by comparing similar populations.
5. Providing credibility for opportunities for change.
6. Helping to provide a view that extends beyond the immediate boundaries.

Source: Adapted from Mulcahy K. Management of diabetes education programs. In: Franz MJ, ed. A Core Curriculum for Diabetes Education: Diabetes Education and Program Management. 5th ed. Chicago: American Association of Diabetes Educators; 2003:208.

Table 2.2  Sample CQI Measures

| Measure | The Joint Commission | DSME Program | Clinic or Institution Specific | Process |
|---|---|---|---|---|
| QC frequency of BG equipment used in hospital or OP setting every 8 hr with signature of trained person doing QC | | | X | X |
| Documentation of home instructions for what patient is to do | | X | | X |
| CPR cart/portable defibrillator for clinics (rationale: risk for heart disease related to DM) | | | X | X |
| Protocol for 911 emergencies | X | | X | X |
| Nurse call lights in each exam room and bathroom | X | | X | X |
| Temperature log on medication/reagent/patient refrigerators | X | | | X |
| Urine ketone testing if BG >250 mg/dL for T1DM | | X | X | X |
| Annual microalbuminuria test documented | | X | | X |
| Referral for annual dilated eye exam documented | | X | | X |
| Foot exam documentation | | X | | X |
| Tobacco cessation counseling | | X | | X |
| Dental exam documentation | | X | | X |
| Cardiac risk reduction meds for individuals with hx of CVD | | X | X | X |
| Patient no-show rate | | X | | X |
| Loss to follow-up rate | | X | | X |

**Table 2.2  Sample CQI Measures** *(Continued)*

| Measure | The Joint Commission | DSME Program | Clinic or Institution Specific | Process |
|---|---|---|---|---|
| Time frame of best-attended education session | | X | | X |
| Exercise prescription | | X | | X |
| Referral to support group or community lifestyle resource | | X | | X |
| Frequency of family attending class | | X | | X |
| Medication change | | | X | X |
| Patient/participant satisfaction with the education program | | X | | X |
| Treatment of hyperglycemia documented, including repeat BG after administration of insulin | | | X | X |
| Adherence of staff to hypoglycemia treatment protocol | | | X | X |
| Adherence of staff to hyperglycemia treatment protocol | | | X | X |
| New form used correctly | | | | X |
| Documentation of behavior goal setting | | X | | X |
| Documentation of behavior goal achievement | | X | | X |
| A1C stratified (<6.5, >9.5, etc.) pre and post program | | X | | X |
| Environment of care indicators met at DSME location | | | X | X |

## Health Status Outcomes and CQI: What's the Difference?

As you are thinking about potential CQI projects, it is important to remember that *outcomes alone do not equal CQI*. In the classic Donabedian Model, outcomes are "a measureable product and . . . the changed state or condition of an individual as a consequence of health care over time."[48] As discussed in this guide, CQI is an ongoing process that affects a broader population in a program. For example, individual patient outcomes are changes in A1C, weight, or LDL-cholesterol, while aggregate population outcomes are the percentage of patients who have both pre- and post-A1C measures and the percentage of participants in an education program who are hospitalized for ketoacidosis.

Standard 10 of the NSDSME/S may help clarify the difference between outcomes and CQI[45]:

> Outcome measures indicate the result of a process (ie, whether changes are actually leading to improvement), while process measures provide information about what caused those results. Process measures are often targeted to those processes that typically affect the most important outcomes.

From the time of the initial intake or assessment to the time of discharge or termination, you are always collecting and reviewing data on the patient's outcomes. You may quantify how much knowledge and skill the person has acquired, what behavior or activity the person is doing, and clinical values and economic impact figures. In contrast, the patient's A1C values, blood pressure readings, type and frequency of activity, missed days from work, normal activities, and visits to the emergency room for problems with blood glucose control are all examples of patient outcome measures.

The CQI process provides staff with methods to find out if patients are achieving outcomes that are appropriate as required by Standard 10 of the NSDSME/S. If not, you must determine whether a program process is contributing to the results or needs improvement. For example, consider a program in which patients currently walk an average of 2,200 steps per day. The goal, however, is 10,000 steps based on patient profile and expressed interest. A CQI process is applied to identify various reasons why patients are not achieving their personal goal(s) as a result of attending an education program. To improve program outcomes, an intervention is planned to support and help patients achieve their desired goals as a result of having attended the program.

## Program and Patient Benefits of CQI

The CQI process can provide important benefits for both your program and your patients. Your diabetes program can benefit in one or more of the following ways:

- Measures the value of your diabetes education service against your organization's mission or your community's needs
- Provides for a systematic, coordinated, and ongoing approach for improving performance that is effectively communicated within your department, organization, or community
- Identifies high-risk patients

- Determines the best way to adhere to local, state, and federal regulatory and reimbursement policies
- Identifies processes or practice guidelines that will improve patient care
- Provides economic information for the healthcare system
- Gathers data to inform the payer of the effectiveness of the program
- Measures the productivity of your program (e.g., staff appointment hours/day, or number of visits to complete treatment or education)

Your patients with diabetes can benefit in one or more of the following ways:

- Increases patient satisfaction
- Decreases waiting times at the healthcare practice setting
- Improves turnaround time for services (e.g., how long it takes to get an appointment or get into a class)
- Matches services offered to community needs (e.g., Does your program offer the volume and types of services appropriate for your community demographics?)
- Avoids or reduces laboratory or diagnostic testing errors (e.g., transcription errors of A1C results during documentation)
- Avoids adverse incidents (e.g., medication errors in prescribing or recommending, or patient self-administration errors)
- Improves patient outcomes in quality of life, following the prescribed treatment plan, and knowledge of diabetes and care requirements
- Reduces the number of unscheduled physician visits related to diabetes
- Reduces the number of emergency room visits related to diabetes
- Improves patient action related to the seven self-care behaviors (Figure 2.1) identified in the AADE position statement *AADE7 Self-Care Behaviors™*.[49]

**Figure 2.1  AADE7 Self-Care Behaviors™**

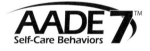

- Healthy Eating
- Being Active
- Monitoring
- Taking Medication
- Problem Solving
- Healthy Coping
- Reducing Risks

# Chapter 3  The CQI Process

All of the various models or systems for guiding quality improvement efforts have certain steps in common, even if the steps have different names. The CQI process described in this book uses the eight steps of CQI as originally described in a technical review, *Diabetes Self-Management Education Core Outcome Measures*.[50] These steps will serve as a guide to clearly delineate all aspects of the CQI process and assist you in meeting your CQI goals. The eight steps described in this chapter are:

1. Identify the Problem/Opportunity
2. Collect the Data
3. Analyze the Data
4. Identify Alternative Solutions
5. Develop an Implementation Plan
6. Implement the Plan
7. Evaluate the Actions
8. Maintain the Improvement

## Before Beginning a CQI Project

You may find it helpful to consider the following points before beginning a CQI project:

1. Collecting data or outcomes is not a CQI effort by itself.
2. CQI projects should be purposeful and based on what is important to you and your program; they should not be done just for the sake of having a record of improvement efforts. Be creative in the projects you choose and how you conduct them.
3. It is not necessary to measure A1C values in all CQI projects. Select projects that can have an impact on the issues affecting your program.
4. Be sure that you have an environment in place that encourages successful collaboration among team members.

### Selecting the CQI Team Members

Before initiating a CQI program, it may be necessary to evaluate staff perceptions of the work environment in areas essential to the success of implementing the recommendations suggested by the CQI project. It is also essential to have a culture or develop one that encourages change through open communication and feedback. The American Health Care Association's *CQI Climate Survey Report Generator* has a 25-statement tool that can be used to identify potential barriers to collaboration on your team that could have a negative impact on the success of your CQI project.[51]

Once a relevant CQI project has been identified, select the appropriate people for your team. A well-balanced team is critical to the success of your CQI efforts. The scope of the project will determine the size, composition, and representation of the CQI team. Choose team members who see the need for CQI and will support the process. Be sure that the team includes members who are familiar with all parts of the CQI process, including those who know the customers and understand their expectations.[52]

You will most likely need to involve staff from outside your immediate education program. Engaging other healthcare professionals in your CQI efforts provides an excellent opportunity to learn and benefit from their expertise. Some organizations have quality or performance improvement departments that can take the lead in designing and implementing a CQI project. If your organization does not have such a department, it is still important to seek participation from outside your immediate program so you are connected to larger organizational goals.

The CQI team should include the following key members:

- System Leader: an individual in a leadership role who has enough authority in the organization to institute a change and overcome barriers that arise. This person must have authority in all areas that are affected by the change and must be able to allocate the time and resources that the team needs to achieve the CQI goal.
- Provider Champion: an individual who has clinical and technical expertise and is familiar with the CQI problem. This expert can provide additional technical support by helping the team determine what to measure, how to measure it, and how to work with the data.
- Data Collection and Analysis Team Member: an individual who manages the data that you wish to collect. You will need to work with this person to obtain the data that you need for your CQI project and to be sure that the data are in a format that is usable for your purposes. The data analysis expert may or may not be the same person who manages the data you are collecting.
- Project Leader: an individual who oversees the day-to-day project activities. This person must understand the details of the problem being studied, as well as the various effects of making changes that are recommended.
- Additional team members as needed, depending on the type of project and the barriers to be overcome. These may include office staff, medical assistants, a nurse, a pharmacist, a dietitian, community health workers, and information system staff.

Use the *Application to Your Practice Worksheet 3.1: CQI Team Candidates* in Appendix III to help you identify potential team members.

## Reporting

Another important part of the quality process to consider before beginning your project is reporting. Information must be passed throughout the chain of command for the process to work well. Leadership and staff must work in concert to ensure that decisions are based on data. These decisions need to be communicated and implemented effectively. Committees that are responsible for quality improvement efforts must keep detailed minutes of meetings, noting action plans that are based on the data. These minutes provide a way to track progress toward quality goals, as well as provide evidence to regulatory agencies that a quality program is active and guiding improvements.

Use the *Application to Your Practice Worksheet 3.2: Project Reporting Form* in Appendix III to help you capture and communicate information on the project.

## Data Collection

Data collection is a form of reporting. To most efficiently collect data, the team must first agree on how the data will be collected. **Do not collect more complex data than is necessary to complete your project.** When collecting data from an electronic medical record (EMR), it is wise to involve someone from the information technology staff to make sure your data can be properly and safely extracted from the EMR. Data collected by paper and/or electronically must be safely stored in a secure location, with electronic data being encrypted on a computer.

## Establishing a Timeline

Quality improvement is sometimes thought to be a long and cumbersome process. In reality, the length of time to complete a CQI project depends on several factors and will vary with each project based on the:

- nature of the project
- ease and ability of collecting and analyzing the data
- time needed to plan, implement, and evaluate the process improvement

When you choose your project, think of the span of time that will give you a snapshot of all of the potential issues. That period might be anywhere from days to months to years, depending on factors such as the amount of data, the scope of the problem, and the number of staff available to work on the project. Allow appropriate time to complete each of the eight steps of the CQI process and to make an informed decision about the change and results.

Program managers should estimate the time points for data collection so proper investments can be made in the technical systems and/or staff processes that can realistically capture the needed information. Most CQI programs will collect data for several months before reviewing the data and making any changes in processes. Ideally, documentation should take place more frequently to identify aggregate level trends in a program evaluation. Outcomes related to the AADE7 Self-Care Behaviors™ can, for example, be documented at baseline (i.e., first visit or class) and then at specified time points, such as months 1, 3, 6, and 12. As part of the protocol, the practice should determine the most effective way to obtain this information based on the practice's patient population. Methods could include face-to-face visits, group classes, mail, e-mail, phone, web conferencing, online surveys, and mobile apps. The key is to document the information with a standardized method. If the information is to be used as part of an overall diabetes program evaluation strategy, this will enable the practice to track the same information at these specified time points so data can be aggregated and reviewed with the instructional staff and advising groups. One approach to doing this is to identify one team member to lead this process. This individual then would manage the process and be responsible for auditing the process, reporting to the group on the process status and milestones, and helping guide the process. If resources permit, managers should consider automating or outsourcing difficult methods of process data collection. For example, the number of participants seen by the diabetes educators, as well as the type of interventions used, could be automatically exported from EMRs into convenient reports.

Building on the background of the development of the CQI processes in general, CQI and its application in the US healthcare sector, and CQI's relationship to DSME, and keeping in mind the considerations just discussed, you and your team are ready to work through the eight steps that are universal to the CQI process and apply them to your own CQI project.

## Step 1: Identify the Problem or Opportunity

The problem or opportunity for improvement first must be identified. It should relate to an opportunity to improve your program or solve an existing problem. Potential CQI projects can be identified from multiple sources, such as program evaluations, verbal comments, audits and inspections, customer data, staff concerns, care plans, or comparisons of external performance benchmarks. Be careful to distinguish between CQI projects and outcomes measurements. (See Table 3.1.)

You and your team may have identified several problems or opportunities that could be addressed. How many of these should you address? You will need as many CQI processes as are necessary to achieve the goals you have established for your patients and your program. Remember that CQI is an ongoing activity that focuses on constant improvement. Please don't confuse what is required for achieving accreditation or recognition status (minimum of one process) with what is needed to improve your program (ongoing, multiple if needed). To help you and your team decide which projects to address, complete the *Application to Your Practice Worksheet 3.3: Potential CQI Projects* in Appendix III. The sample CQI project box below (Sample CQI Project 3.1) will be used throughout the remainder of this guide to demonstrate the eight steps of the CQI process.

---

**Sample CQI Project 3.1**

**Problem:** Patients and providers complain about how long it takes to get into the diabetes education classes (appointment delay problem)

**Goal:** Ensure that patients receive timely access to diabetes education classes

---

**Table 3.1  CQI and Outcome Measures**

| Potential CQI Project | **Not Recommended for CQI Projects (These are outcomes measurements, not CQI)** *Type of measure or activity indicated in parentheses following description.* |
|---|---|
| Increase the percentage of program participants walking 10,000 steps per day | Gathering data and reporting on the number of program participants who chose physical activity/ exercises (behavior change objective) and how many achieve their goals (behavior change objective) |
| Increase the number of program participants who are referred for counseling for depression | Screening program participants for depression (clinical activity) |
| Increase the number of program participants who do foot self-exams | Gathering data and reporting on the number of program participants who perform a foot self-exam (program outcome measure) Studying whether program participants who have had a negative foot exam have changed their foot care behavior (research) |
| Increase the number of program participants who have pre-program and post-program A1C lab results | Gathering data and reporting on the number of program participants who have pre-program and post-program A1C results (program outcome measure) |
| Improve participant follow-up in the education program | Gathering data and reporting on how many program participants complete the comprehensive program through the follow-up portion of the program (program data) |
| Decrease no-show rate for appointments | Gathering data and reporting on how many program participants do not cancel their appointments and do not show up for their appointments (program data) |
| Improve the reimbursement for program services | Gathering information on the actual reimbursement for program participants (program data) |
| Improve staff efficiency | Having the staff keep time studies on productive and nonproductive time (program data) |

## Step 2: Collect the Data

One of the strengths of CQI is that it is based on facts and data. Quality improvement efforts that are supported by data are more likely to produce real improvements than efforts not based on such research.

During this step, your CQI team gathers data on suspected problems and operations, such as issues that caused the problems and barriers to solving them. It is important for the team to use the CQI process to identify and analyze potential causes of the problems or barriers to improvement. One simple way to collect such information is to give all team members a pad of sticky notes and ask them to write as many different possible causes of the problem as they can, using one note for each problem. These notes can then be placed on a flip chart for viewing. Omit duplicate ideas, group similar ideas, and add other ideas as they emerge during the discussion. An affinity diagram is an example of this technique. (See Figure 3.1.)

Another tool that provides a visual representation of data is a fishbone diagram, which is used to show cause and effect. This type of diagram gives a visual representation of the various causes that contribute to a single effect and can help your CQI team explore the possible causes of a given problem. Figure 3.2 illustrates a simple fishbone diagram showing possible causes of the appointment delay problem.

**Figure 3.1  Sample Affinity Diagram**

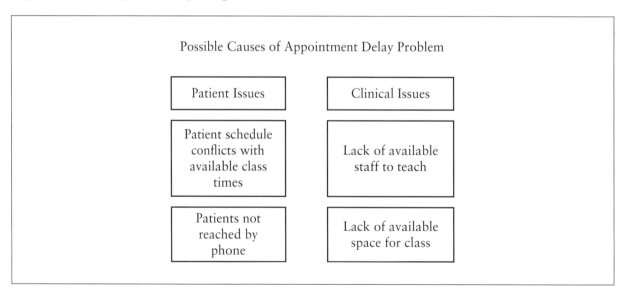

**Figure 3.2  Sample Fishbone Diagram**

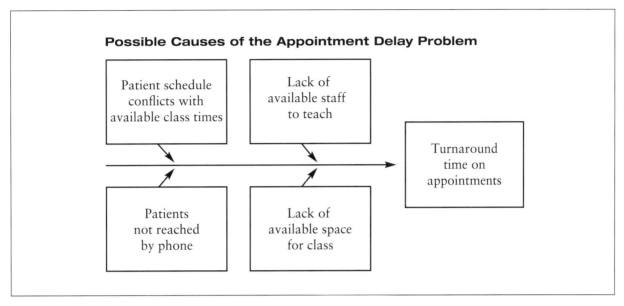

After determining the possible issues related to your CQI project, data need to be gathered on these issues. Data can be categorized into one of 3 levels of measurement:

1. *Variable data*, also called interval data, are quantified numeric data stated in standard units of measures, for example, how many, how much, how far, number of minutes waiting, ounces of fluid consumed, and so forth. Variable data offer the greatest range of possibilities for analysis.
2. *Ordinal data* have been quantified using non-numeric standards such as in the Likert scales, for example, 5 = very satisfied, 4 = somewhat satisfied, 3 = satisfied, and so forth.
3. *Attribute data*, also called nominal data, are categorical data such as sex, race, religion, admitted/not admitted, and so forth.[53]

Data can be collected from across the healthcare continuum:

- Clinical outcomes
- Health status outcomes
- Quality-of-life (QOL) outcomes
- Behavioral outcomes
- Patient-centered outcomes
- Cost outcomes
- Cost effectiveness
- Cost benefit
- Program outcomes
- Process measures

Identify what data to collect and a specific time frame for the data to be collected. The tools used to collect the data depend on the problem identified or the process to be improved. Table 3.2 highlights some data collection tools.

**Table 3.2  Data Collection Tools**

| Method | Examples of Outcomes Collected | Easy to Use? | Yields Reliable Data? | High Response Rate? |
|---|---|---|---|---|
| *Survey:* Method used to question individuals in writing, face-to-face, by phone, or by mail | Learning; behavior change; quality of life; satisfaction | Yes. Can be designed to be simple and easy to use. | Yes, although respondents' interpretation of survey questions can vary. | Depends. Telephone or face-to-face surveys can have a high response rate. |
| *Chart/File Audit:* Review of closed, open, or computerized medical records to retrieve information | Lab data (A1C, lipids); process data (eye or foot exam) | Depends. Paper chart review can be labor-intensive and time-intensive. | Depends on skill of individuals doing the review. | Yes |
| *Checklist:* Data collection sheet for gathering concurrent information during a study | Behavior change; process and implementation tasks | Yes. Can be designed to be simple and easy to use | Depends. All people who will be completing the checklist during the data collection must be trained on how to use the data collection instrument. | Depends on the cooperation and availability of the personnel completing the forms. |
| *Time Study:* Concurrent formation about time to complete a process such as turnaround time | Cycle time to schedule a patient for a visit | Usually very time-intensive and labor-intensive | Depends. All people who will be completing the time study during the data collection must be trained on how to use the instrument. | Depends on the cooperation and availability of the personnel completing the study. |
| *Interview:* Method used to question individuals face-to-face or by phone, online survey, or mobile app | People's attitudes, beliefs, behavior, health status, satisfaction, needs, or expectations | Face-to-face or phone usually very time-intensive and labor-intensive; online or mobile app easy for user. Depending on the tool, can require technical skills to build and support | Depends. All people who will be conducting the interview during the data collection must be trained on how to use the instrument and how to interview people. For online and mobile, are self-report with limitations on follow-up questions. | Depends on the cooperation and availability of the personnel completing the study. For online and mobile, depends on Internet access. |

Source: Adapted from Mulcahy K. Management of diabetes education programs. In: Franz MJ, ed. A Core Curriculum for Diabetes Educators. 5th ed. Chicago, IL: American Association of Diabetes Educators; 2003:203.

Before developing a data collection plan, ensure that your program is in compliance with the Health Insurance Portability and Accountability Act (HIPAA) privacy rules on protecting health information. Sample CQI Project 3.2 illustrates a data collection tool used for the sample CQI project on the appointment delay problem. Data were collected from 85 patients; however, the table reflects data from only 4 patients.

**Sample CQI Project 3.2**

## Data Collection Tool for the Appointment Delay Problem

| Patient ID No. | Date of Patient Call | Date of Returned Call | Date of 1st Available Appt. | Actual Appt. Date | Reason for Delay* | Total Days† |
|---|---|---|---|---|---|---|
| 1 | 4/1 | 4/15 | 6/15 | -- | c | NA |
| 2 | 4/2 | 4/4 | 6/8 | 7/30 | c | 114 |
| 3 | 4/3 | 4/15 | 6/15 | 8/15 | e | 134 |
| 85 | 4/30 | 4/30 | 6/30 | 6/30 | d | 6 |

Data collection period from April 1 through April 30.
*Reason code:
a—Patient schedule conflicts with available class time.
b—Lack of available staff to teach.
c—Patient not reached by phone.
d—Lack of available space for class.
e—Other (record reason, such as vacation).
† Total days from initial phone call by patient until the class date that the patient was scheduled to attend.

It is important to determine an appropriate sample size so your study population provides a good representation of the problem being studied. Table 3.3 is an example of a "look-up" sample size chart that will tell you how many charts to include in your sample, depending on how many patients you have in your eligible population. This chart is based on a sample size calculated for a 95% confidence interval. In many instances, it may be simpler to include your entire patient population.

If you are unable to easily generate a random list of charts to review by patient or enrollment number, there is a simple way to identify the patients to be included in your sample. Divide the total number of eligible patients you have identified in your register(s) or active case list by the

Table 3.3  Look-up Sample Size Chart

| Population Size | Sample Size | Population Size | Sample Size |
|---|---|---|---|
| Up to 20 | All | 160-179 | 82 |
| 30 | 26 | 180-199 | 86 |
| 40 | 32 | 200-249 | 94 |
| 50 | 38 | 250-299 | 101 |
| 60 | 43 | 300-349 | 106 |
| 70 | 48 | 350-399 | 110 |
| 80 | 53 | 400-449 | 113 |
| 90 | 57 | 450-499 | 116 |
| 100 | 61 | 500-749 | 127 |
| 101-119 | 67 | 750-999 | 131 |
| 120-139 | 73 | 1,000-4,999 | 146 |
| 140-159 | 78 | 5,000 or more | 150 |

Note: Sample size calculated for a 95% confidence interval with a width of 0.16, based on a predicted score of 50%.

Source: Chapter 11, Quality improvement. In: Operations Manual for Delivery of HIV Prevention, Care and Treatment at Primary Health Centres in High-Prevalence, Resource-Constrained Settings. World Health Organization; 2008.

number of patients you need to review, based on the information in Table 3.3. You will use this number to create the sequence of your sample. For example, if you have 750 eligible patients for referrals for counseling for depression, the look-up table tells you that your sample should be 131. If you divide 750 by 131, the result is 6. You will now need to take your ordered list (or patient cards arranged in order of enrollment) and select every sixth patient. The list you use has to be one that records each patient only once.[54]

## Step 3: Analyze the Data

During this step, your team reviews and analyzes the data that were collected. Responses obtained from the data collection tool can be tallied in a simple table format or entered into a spreadsheet program and displayed as a *time series graph* or *run chart*. An example of the sample CQI project data is shown in Sample CQI Project 3.3. Organizing the data in these formats facilitates making key observations. Consider some basic questions, such as:

- What are the main problems?
- Are there any results that were unexpected?

---

**Sample CQI Project 3.3**

**Data Analysis of Causes of Appointment Delay**

Baseline data: Average turnaround time was 60 days.

| Code | Reason | Responses n (%) |
|------|--------|-----------------|
| a | Patient schedule conflicts with available class times | 20 (20) |
| b | Lack of available staff to teach | 5 (5) |
| c | Patients not reached by phone | 15 (15) |
| d | Lack of available space for class | 45 (45) |
| e | Other (note reason) | 15 (15) |

---

At this point in the process, unanticipated problems may be revealed and may require a separate CQI project. Your CQI team will need to prioritize the problems to determine which one to address first. Complete documentation of the data collection and analysis steps will provide a record that may be useful for later referral. In addition, it is important to communicate the results of the data analysis to decision makers in the organization to gain their support and assistance with project planning.

Another way to analyze the data is to present the results in a *Pareto* data table and diagram. The *Pareto Principle* is that relatively few factors account for the majority of the effects. Presenting the information in a Pareto diagram will help the team identify the factors that have the greatest impact and communicate the results to others. The data are first organized into a Pareto chart (Table 3.4) that can then be converted into a graph by entering the data into a spreadsheet program (Figure 3.3). In the example, the data are presented from the highest to lowest frequency in percent as well as cumulative percent.

**Table 3.4  Data Analysis of Causes of Appointment Delay**

| Reason | Percent | Cumulative Percent |
|---|---|---|
| Lack of available space for class | 45 | 45 |
| Patient schedule conflicts with available class times | 20 | 65 |
| Patients not reached by phone | 15 | 80 |
| Other (note reason) | 15 | 95 |
| Lack of available staff to teach | 5 | 100 |

**Figure 3.3  Pareto Chart**

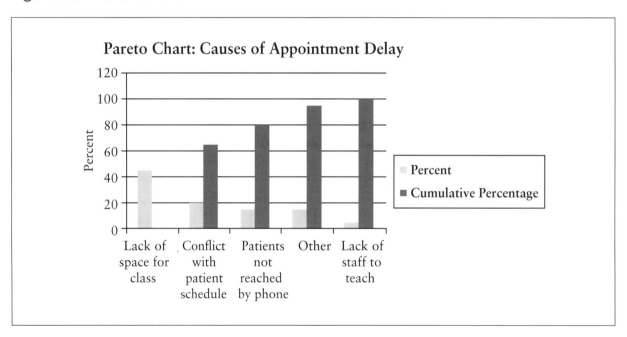

By reviewing the Pareto chart it is easy to see that 3 factors accounted for 80% of the causes of the appointment delay. To help you plan your data analysis, answer the questions on *Application to Your Practice Worksheet 3.4: Data Collection for Your CQI Project* in Appendix III. For additional information on data analysis tools and methods, see Appendix II.

What else can you do with the information and data that you've collected? The information should be used to make decisions about your program and processes. But don't let it stop there. Use the information to market your program.

In the Sample CQI Project regarding the appointment delay problem, you could promote your program by placing a flyer at the appointment desk claiming better customer service with more available appointments. In your brochure, you could highlight the availability of evening classes and larger classroom space.

You should always report results concerning the project and process to the oversight/advisory committee of your program.

## Step 4: Identify Alternative Solutions

Now that you've analyzed the data, your team can begin to identify changes that will result in improvement, and then develop opportunities and strategies to improve specific processes or solve specific problems. This step provides an opportunity to exercise creative thinking. One way of identifying alternative solutions is to use *brainstorming,* a method of generating many free-flowing ideas without discussion or judgment. Some brainstorming results for the appointment delay problem are shown in Sample CQI Project 3.4.

---

**Sample CQI Project 3.4**

**Brainstorming Results for the Appointment Delay Problem\***
**Possible Solutions**

- Ask administration for a larger room
- Hold classes at the local library or community center
- Apply for an NIH building grant
- Hold virtual classes
- Purchase smaller table to make more room for chairs
- Hold classes in the office of largest referral service
- Hold classes in the lobby area after hours

\*Delay due to lack of space available.

---

There are two types of brainstorming, *unstructured* and *structured.* With unstructured brainstorming, team members give ideas as fast as they come to mind, and all ideas are recorded by a designated person. With structured brainstorming, team members write down their ideas and then take turns offering one idea at a time. For both forms of brainstorming, there is no limit to the number of ideas that can be offered and no discussion of the ideas. It is important to make a list of all suggested solutions because you never know when a seemingly unusual idea will turn into a dynamic creative solution that meets everyone's needs in unanticipated ways.

When choosing optimal change strategies, the following factors should be considered:

- Clinical importance
- Cost/benefit ratio
- Time/benefit ratio
- Effectiveness
- Feasibility of implementing
- Shortest timeline
- Solution to the root cause
- Acceptability to those most affected

The results of the team discussion on alternative solutions are shown in Sample CQI Project 3.5.

---

**Sample CQI Project 3.5**

**Identify Alternative Solutions for the Appointment Delay Problem**

When all possible solutions were discussed, the team decided to choose the solution that was the least costly and easiest to implement—to ask the administration for an appropriate room space.

The team developed a plan to test whether increasing the size of the room would allow more participants in each class and thus improve the appointment turnaround time.

---

## Step 5: Develop an Implementation Plan

This step involves planning how to apply the change. The following basic questions can be used to guide your implementation plan:

- Who is going to be involved?
- What is going to be changed?
- When will this happen?
- Where will this take place?
- Why did we choose to test this solution?
- How are we going to do it?

Good communication about the implementation plan with all who are involved or who will be affected will encourage their commitment to the proposed change. An effective way to keep all team members informed is to prepare a written plan that identifies the specific steps of the solution and designates the persons responsible for each step or task (Sample CQI Project 3.6). The implementation plan should also include a time frame for testing the solution. The team might find it necessary to test several solutions or improvement processes. However, test only one solution at a time so you can accurately evaluate its impact.

**Sample CQI Project 3.6**

**Implementation Plan**

| Action Plan | Responsible Person |
|---|---|
| 1. Team meets to discuss new schedule | Diabetes program director |
| 2. Scheduler is notified that class size will increase to 10 participants effective July 1 | Day-to-day project leader |
| 3. Number of patient slots is increased in the database | Scheduler |
| 4. Patients who have appointments after July 1 are notified of the availability of class at an earlier date | Scheduler |
| 5. Time frame is established to reassess turnaround time | CQI team |

# Step 6: Implement the Plan

Step 6 involves testing the change in an actual practice setting while observing the results and collecting data. The amount of time required to implement the plan will vary depending on factors such as the complexity of the plan, the number of participants, availability of the space, and so forth. All team members must receive specific in-service training on the implementation plan, including details of the starting date. Continuous communication and reinforcement are essential for successful implementation. (See Sample CQI Project 3.7.)

**Sample CQI Project 3.7**

**Implement a Plan for the Appointment Delay Problem**

A new, larger space was made available on July 1. The same data collection tool that was used in Step 2 was used during the implementation step to collect data for 90 days to evaluate the impact of the solution.

## Step 7: Evaluate the Actions

At the end of the specific time frame your team chose for implementing and tracking the action plan developed in Steps 5 and 6, your CQI team should evaluate the results of the implemented changes. Because various data have been collected throughout the implementation step, compilation of the data for analysis should be a relatively easy task. If the evaluation reveals that the implemented plan did not achieve the desired result, Steps 4 through 7 *should be repeated* with a different solution until a satisfactory improvement has been achieved. (See Sample CQI Project 3.8.)

---

### Sample CQI Project 3.8

**Evaluate the Plan for the Appointment Delay Problem**

Data analysis revealed that making a larger space available for the diabetes education classes improved the turnaround time for attending the class (average turnaround time = 45 days).

Lack of available slots in current class times accounted for 35% of delayed appointments, and patient conflict with scheduled classes accounted for 30% of delayed appointments.

After some improvements, the CQI team decided to address the problem of patient schedule conflicts. The solution they chose was to schedule alternative class times, such as evenings and weekends.

---

## Step 8: Maintain the Improvement

Once the improvement has been tested and proved successful, periodic evaluation should be performed. The findings should then be reported to any strategic planning or advisory committee that oversees the program. A *histogram* is an effective tool for providing a visual comparison of progress over time. An example of a display of data and maintaining improvement can be seen in Sample CQI Project 3.9. This figure displays the appointment turnaround time from baseline to 12 months after implementing the CQI project. The reduction in turnaround time for appointments resulted in more patients attending class (Sample CQI Project 3.10).

**Sample CQI Project 3.9**

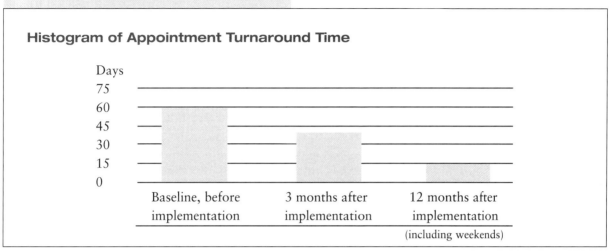

**Histogram of Appointment Turnaround Time**

Days

75
60
45
30
15
0

Baseline, before implementation

3 months after implementation

12 months after implementation

(including weekends)

**Sample CQI Project 3.10**

After a year of CQI efforts, the appointment turnaround time was improved by acquiring additional space and offering alternative times for the diabetes education classes. The additional classes were added to the program brochure to inform the community of the greater accessibility to the diabetes education program services.

To see the Sample CQI Project organized in a chart with all eight steps of the CQI process, see Sample CQI Project 3.11 at the end of this chapter.

What have you learned from this CQI project that you can apply to future projects? Immediately following a CQI project cycle is a good time to note where your DSME program stands, what problems or issues would be the next CQI project to implement, or what changes you would make in utilizing the process or in the composition of your CQI team.

To begin capturing information for your next CQI project, complete *Application to Your Practice Worksheet 3.5: The CQI Process and Its Applications to Your Practice* in Appendix III.

## Sample CQI Project 3.11

### CQI Process for the Appointment Delay Problem, Steps 1 Through 4

| Step 1. Identify the Problem/ Opportunity | Patients and providers complain about how long it takes to get into diabetes education classes. CQI team is formed, consists of program coordinator, scheduler, coordinator/educator, and 3 representatives (registration, billing, CQI) |
|---|---|
| Step 2. Collect the Data | Team uses fishbone diagram to identify all possible causes of appointment delay problem:<br>• Patient schedule conflict<br>• Lack of staff<br>• Lack of space<br>• Patients not reached by phone<br>Data collection tool created (see Table 3.2) to tabulate patient calls and reasons for delay<br>Time frame set at 30 days |
| Step 3. Analyze the Data | Average turnaround time for diabetes class >60 days<br>Top 2 reasons for appointment delays:<br>• 45% due to lack of class space (see Table 3.4)<br>• 20% due to patient schedule conflicts with available classes |
| Step 4. Identify Alternative Solutions | Brainstorming results:<br>• Ask for larger classroom<br>• Offer classes at offsite location<br>• Identify alternative methods of providing education<br>• Use smaller tables to make space for more participants<br>• Hold classes in lobby after hours<br>Team decides to ask for access to a larger room (least costly and easiest option to pursue first) |

**CQI Process for the Appointment Delay Problem, Steps 5 Through 8**

| | |
|---|---|
| **Step 5.** Develop an Implementation Plan | • Expand classes to accommodate 10 patients per class<br>• Set up new class schedule<br>• Inform scheduler that maximum class size increased to 10<br>• Increase number of patient slots in appointment database<br>• Set time frame to evaluate changes on turnaround time |
| **Step 6.** Implement the Plan | Complete all items in Step 5 |
| **Step 7.** Evaluate the Actions | Results 3 months after implementing larger class size:<br>• Turnaround time decreased from 60 days to 45 days<br>• 35% of delayed appointments due to lack of available class slots<br>• 30% due to patient schedule conflicts with available classes<br>Team decides to work on alternative class times |
| **Step 8.** Maintain the Improvement | Results 12 months after implementing larger class size and offering alternative times:<br>• Turnaround time decreased from 60 days to 15 days<br>• No complaints from patients or providers regarding appointment delays<br>• Diabetes Advisory Committee, administration informed of CQI project and results |

## Making Your CQI Project *Stick*

After you have successfully completed the CQI process, your quality improvement project hasn't ended—your commitment to providing the best care possible for people with diabetes is a journey. It is necessary and helpful to have periodical evaluations, but also keep in mind the following tips:

- Step back from the details of the project and take a look at the larger problem. Remind both yourself and your teammates why this is important and why the culture needs to adopt quality improvement.
- Create a culture of self-examination. When reviewing your data at periodic evaluations, ask the hard questions. If the process isn't working, don't be afraid to go back and tweak the protocol.
- Embrace the team approach to working through your CQI problem, and embrace new roles it may bring with it. Although team members may be experts in their field, be open to inviting new team members so that other individuals can learn a new skill set.
- Once you begin to see results, share your improvement journey story. Prepare an elevator speech for those ready and willing to hear your story inside your department, outside your department, and outside your organization. The best way to learn about improvement is to share best practices.

As the work becomes routine in your daily practice, your quality improvement efforts will begin to *stick* and your periodic evaluations will show improvement, allowing you to identify your next CQI project.

# Chapter 4  Case Studies

In this chapter, the eight steps of the CQI process are applied to five cases that represent experiences that might be encountered in a typical DSME program. Note that not all of the cases described below show results that met the CQI goal. Like most DSME programs, some of these cases describe initial CQI projects that generated some improvements, but will require repetition of the process to fully achieve the goal of the project.

## Case 1: Missing A1C Data

The Oversight/Advisory Committee of a DSME program decided to use A1C values as a program outcomes measure. The program coordinator spent several months collecting pre-program and post-program A1C values for participants. The results revealed that many participants did not have these A1C values in their charts. Thus, a problem was identified, requiring CQI intervention (**Step 1**).

The Oversight/Advisory Committee organizes a CQI team to investigate possible reasons for the insufficient A1C data and determine how to improve the data collection process. This team consists of the following members:

- the professional staff of the DSME program
- at least one of the referring physicians or nurse practitioners who make the most referrals to the DSME program
- someone who represents the laboratory
- an office staff person who reviews orders and referrals with patients

The team collects data (**Step 2**) on how many program participants have pre-program and post-program A1C values in their charts. The data are analyzed (**Step 3**) and categorized according to the referral sources. Of the 200 charts reviewed, only 35% have pre-program A1C values and only 25% have post-program A1C values. The referral sources are shown in Table 4.1.

Results of the data analysis show that Provider A's patient referrals do not have pre-program and post-program A1C lab results. To find out why these lab values are missing, one of the team members speaks with Provider A (**Step 3**). Possible reasons for the lack of A1C results are shown in this cause-and-effect diagram or fishbone diagram (Figure 4.1). The team discovers that Provider A actually has the A1C lab values for most of his referrals. However, he did not communicate this information to the DSME program because he was unaware that A1C data were being collected.

As a result of this new information, the team has a brainstorming session (**Step 4**) on how to improve the data collection process so that all of Provider A's patient referrals have pre-program and post-program A1C lab results. The following alternative strategies are identified:

- Revise the referral form to include a space to record A1C values
- Inform all providers of the CQI evaluation being conducted and the importance of sending A1C lab results to the DSME program for all patient referrals

Table 4.1  Referrals

| Provider | Number of Patient Referrals | Number of Pre-Program A1C Values, n (%) | Number of Post-Program A1C Values, n (%) |
|---|---|---|---|
| A | 60 | 0 (0) | 0 (0) |
| B | 40 | 20 (50) | 20 (50) |
| C | 20 | 15 (75) | 5 (25) |
| D | 40 | 15 (38) | 10 (25) |
| E | 20 | 10 (50) | 10 (50) |
| F | 20 | 10 (50) | 5 (25) |
| Total | 200 | 78 (35) | 50 (25) |

Figure 4.1  Possible Reasons for Lack of A1C Data

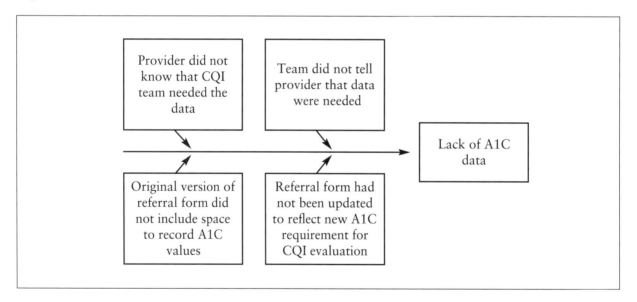

- Mark the calendar to contact Provider A's office for A1C values 3 months after his patient referrals complete the program
- Purchase an A1C analyzer for the DSME program so these lab values can be collected onsite

The alternative solution that was selected to evaluate was revising the referral form. The implementation plan was established (**Step 5**) by including Provider A in this decision and giving his office staff the new referral form to begin using as of a specific date. The CQI team planned to collect data from a chart review for 30 days after Provider A began using the new referral form (**Step 6**). When this action was evaluated, A1C data collection increased to 75% (**Step 7**).

The data were presented to all providers, and they agreed to begin using the new patient referral form. Over the next 6 to 12 months, the program coordinator reported the improvements to the Oversight/Advisory Committee, showing a higher percentage of program participants with both pre-program and post-program A1C lab values. Table 4.2 summarizes the CQI process for Case 1: Missing A1C Data.

**Table 4.2   Case 1: Missing A1C Data. CQI Steps 1 Through 8**

| **Step 1.** Identify the Problem/ Opportunity | • A1C is selected as a program outcomes measure<br>• Many patients do not have both pre-program and post-program A1C test results<br>• A1C values for referred patients are obtained from providers |
|---|---|
| **Step 2.** Collect the Data | Data collected by reviewing patient charts (see Table 4.1 for sample data collection tool) |
| **Step 3.** Analyze the Data | Results show that patient referrals from Provider A were missing A1C data |
| **Step 4.** Identify Alternative Solutions | Brainstorming results:<br>• Revise the referral form to highlight the need for providing A1C values for all patients<br>• Inform all providers of the CQI evaluation being conducted<br>• Mark calendar to remind Provider A's office to send A1C values 3 months after his patients complete the DSME program<br>• Purchase A1C analyzer.<br>Team decides to modify referral form |
| **Step 5.** Develop Implementation Plan | Goal: Obtain pre-program/post-program A1C values for 70% of participants<br>Action Steps:<br>• Revise referral forms to highlight need for A1C lab results for all patients to be sent to DSME program<br>• Distribute revised form to Provider A<br>• Establish a specific starting date for Provider A to begin using new referral form |
| **Step 6.** Implement the Plan | • Track A1C values for Provider A's patients for 30 days after start date<br>• Get referral form to provider<br>• Inform staff in practice where to put A1C value on form<br>• Inform all staff of start date |
| **Step 7.** Evaluate the Actions | Results from tracking A1C data for Provider A's patients showed an increase to 75% in A1C data being provided |

*(continued)*

**Table 4.2   Case 1: Missing A1C Data. CQI Steps 1 Through 8 (continued)**

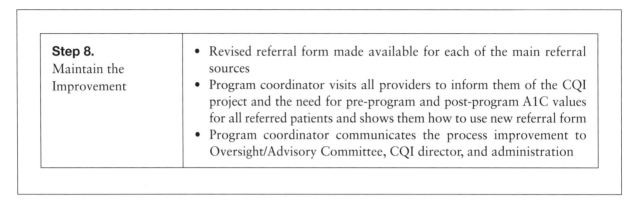

| **Step 8.** Maintain the Improvement | • Revised referral form made available for each of the main referral sources<br>• Program coordinator visits all providers to inform them of the CQI project and the need for pre-program and post-program A1C values for all referred patients and shows them how to use new referral form<br>• Program coordinator communicates the process improvement to Oversight/Advisory Committee, CQI director, and administration |
|---|---|

## Case 2: Measuring Behavior Change

Behavior change can reflect the impact of diabetes education; therefore, it can be worthwhile to focus your CQI efforts on these kinds of projects. (See Figure 4.2.) The direct result of obtaining knowledge and skills through diabetes education can promote behavior change, which will improve clinical parameters and can positively affect the health status of patients. Table 4.3 shows how CQI efforts can be used to improve behavioral outcomes.

**Figure 4.2   Outcomes Continuum**

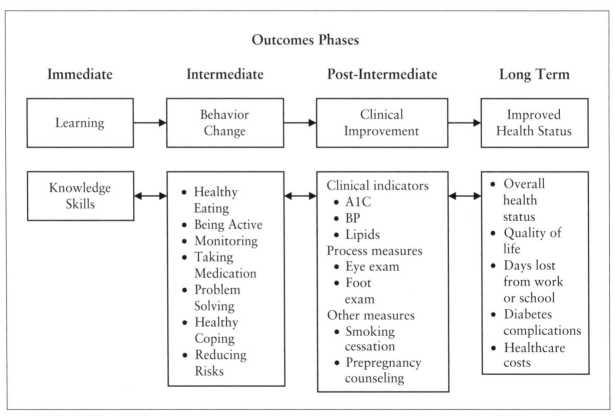

Source: Adapted from Mulcahy K, Maryniuk M, Peeples M, et al. Diabetes self-management education core outcome measures (technical review). *Diabetes Educ.* 2003;29(5):768-803.

**Table 4.3   Case 2: Measuring Behavior Change. CQI Steps 1 Through 8**

| | |
|---|---|
| **Step 1.**<br>Identify the Problem/<br>Opportunity | • Increasing physical activity is selected as a priority goal for the increased health benefit of the patient population<br>• Many program participants are discouraged about achieving their goals<br>• CQI team is formed consisting of educator, exercise specialist, behavioral specialist, and CQI representative |
| **Step 2.**<br>Collect the Data | • Determine what percentage of participants met exercise goal >70% of the time<br>• Determine exercise frequency, type, and duration; barriers to exercising; and A1C population mean |
| **Step 3.**<br>Analyze the Data | CQI team reviews the data and determines that many participants work long hours, have long commutes, and lead sedentary lifestyles.<br><br>• Priority exercise goal 76%<br>• Goal achievement 44%<br>• Exercise frequency <2 days/wk<br>• 30% exercised by walking<br>• Duration <30 min<br>• Barriers were time, environment<br>• Mean A1C value 7.8% |
| **Step 4.**<br>Identify Alternative<br>Solutions | Options from brainstorming:<br><br>• Develop a walking program based on "10,000 steps per day" program<br>• Give each participant a pedometer<br>• Set up a walking club area on organization's website<br>• Give out exercise DVDs<br>• Provide list of local exercise resources<br>• Provide more exercise handouts |
| **Step 5.**<br>Develop<br>Implementation Plan | Team chooses to pilot "10,000 steps" program with 20 participants for 6 months; provides pedometers and activity logs; collects data on goal achievement and barriers at each visit; collects A1C data at baseline and after pilot study |
| **Step 6.**<br>Implement the Plan | Pilot program is implemented with 20 participants who are followed for 6 months |
| **Step 7.**<br>Evaluate the Actions | Results at 6 months: average self-reported goal achievement was 79%; pedometer records showed 6,400 average steps per day; A1C population mean was 6.4%; team decides to implement program for all patients |
| **Step 8.**<br>Maintain the<br>Improvement | Program was implemented for all patients; data 1 year later show goal at 74%, achievement at 68%, frequency at >3x/wk; walking was main type of exercise, duration at <30 min, steps at 6,900/day; A1C population mean at 6.2%; program director communicates process improvement results to Diabetes Advisory Group, administration, and other stakeholders; improved behavioral outcomes added to program brochure |

## Case 3: Improving Turnaround Time

The problem identified was the long wait time for scheduling high-risk patients—those with gestational diabetes or newly diagnosed type 1 diabetes—in a diabetes education program. Table 4.4 shows the steps to improving the turnaround time for the high-risk patients.

**Table 4.4   Case 3: Improving Turnaround Time in a Diabetes Education Program. CQI Steps 1 Through 8**

| | |
|---|---|
| **Step 1.** Identify the Problem/ Opportunity | Improve patient health outcomes by ensuring that high-risk patients are seen quickly and within the community time frame. |
| **Step 2.** Collect the Data | Quarterly turnaround time by site/location and DSME service. |
| **Step 3.** Analyze the Data | A difference of 50-day turnaround time between sites. |
| **Step 4.** Identify Alternative Solutions | Increase staffing hours of educators and establish internal benchmark of 10 days' turnaround time. Collect turnaround time for high-risk and high-volume population before establishing a benchmark for these groups. |
| **Step 5.** Develop Implementation Plan | Updated data collection tool to include type of service needed. Defined emergent visits and established targets for turnaround time for DSME services. Communicated CQI plan to all team members. |
| **Step 6.** Implement the Plan | Collected quarterly data over a 2-week period. Tracked results quarterly by site. |
| **Step 7.** Evaluate the Actions | All program services met targets for turnaround time except for evening classes and visits for patients with newly diagnosed type 1 diabetes. |
| **Step 8.** Maintain the Improvement | Continue to collect quarterly data to obtain baseline data and continue to refine data collection methods. Consider opportunities to increase number of evening classes if the class size continues to interfere with meeting target turnaround time. |

Source: Adapted with permission. Lumber T. Improving turn-around time in a diabetes education program—a CQI case study. *AADE in Practice*. 2007 (Fall):4.

# Case 4: Evaluating Behavior Change Across DSME Sites

In this case study, the focus of the CQI was to evaluate the effectiveness of the DSME program in facilitating behavior change of participants from multiple sites within the same organization. The CQI program identified the behavioral goals most commonly selected by patients, the percentage of patients meeting their goals, and the processes needed to support behavioral goals. Table 4.5 indicates the steps for evaluating the DSME program's behavior change outcomes.

**Table 4.5   Case 4: Improving Program DSME Behavior Change Outcomes. CQI Steps 1 Through 8**

| | |
|---|---|
| **Step 1.** Identify the Problem/ Opportunity | As a multisite diabetes program, how successful are we in helping participants make behavior change? |
| **Step 2.** Collect the Data | What are the most frequently chosen behavior goals by participants with type 2 diabetes attending class? <br><br> By program site? <br><br> What percentage of patients achieved their goals most or all of the time (4 or 5 rating on goal sheet with the highest possible rating of 5)? <br><br> Are we reaching a target of 70% of patients achieving goals? |
| **Step 3.** Analyze the Data | The most frequently selected goal was "being active" and the average goal achievement was 70%. <br><br> The second most frequently selected goal was "healthy eating" and the average goal achievement was 54%. |
| **Step 4.** Identify Alternative Solutions | For "healthy eating" goal: <br> • Improve goal-setting efforts by diabetes educator team <br> • Be consistent in how goals are rated by site <br> • Revise goal-setting worksheet <br> • Provide additional staff training on how to improve behavior change teaching skills <br> • Hire a behavioral expert to help teach the class |
| **Step 5.** Develop Implementation Plan | Check goal-setting worksheet of each participant at the end of class. <br><br> Review "healthy eating" goals of participants to ensure that goals are specific and achievable. |
| **Step 6.** Implement the Plan | Communicate plan with all staff. <br><br> Collect data beginning with the 2nd quarter and evaluate during 3rd and 4th quarters. |

*(continued)*

**Table 4.5  Case 4: Improving Program DSME Behavior Change Outcomes. CQI Steps 1 Through 8 (continued)**

| **Step 7.** Evaluate the Actions | Percentage of participants reaching "healthy eating" goal: 2nd quarter: 55% to 68% 3rd quarter: 65% 4th quarter: 63% |
|---|---|
| **Step 8.** Maintain the Improvement | Repeat the PDSA cycle by identifying another solution: Achieve consistent rating of goals at all 3 program sites. |

Source: Adapted from presentation by Terry Lumber, RN, CNS, MSN, CDE, BC, ADM, The Use of CQI to Improve DSMT Program Outcomes: Describe How the CQI Process Can Improve Program Outcomes.

## Case 5: Follow-Up of High-Risk Patients

This case study provides a real-life example of a scenario that all types of providers encounter within their career: better follow-up of high-risk patients. In this example, which is explained in PDSA format, the CQI team is specifically targeting patients with an A1C >9 who did not keep suggested follow-up appointments within the past year. In order to uncover the problem, the team performed the following PDSA cycle:

**Plan:** Select a provider who is willing and able to champion the idea. Pull the provider's patient panel and associated data (A1C, follow-up appointments, contact information) and identify patients that fit the criteria.

**Do:** Create a tracking sheet (Word®, Excel®) to track patients and barriers to them making their appointments. Contact patients that meet the above criteria by phone, secure portal messaging, or mail and track the reasons why they did not keep their suggested appointments. If the patients wanted to reschedule an appointment or had another issue, such as an outstanding bill, the office assistant could help them while they were on the phone. Track outcomes of the conversation.

**Study:** Analyze the data. What percentage of patients had outstanding bills? What percentage of patients didn't have transportation? What percentage of patients were no longer patients, e.g., transferred care?

**Act:** Meet with the rest of the CQI team and share your results. Based on the analysis of your data, come up with ideas on how to fix the most important problems. In this case, the CQI team investigated having an automatic phone messaging system call patients if they missed appointments and/or if they didn't schedule one. Due to contact issues, the CQI team also decided to have "lapse patient letters" scheduled to go out to patients sooner than a year for reminders.

The PDSA cycle for learning and improvement (see Figure 4.3) model has two parts: three questions that help set the change for improvement and then the PDSA cycle, which allows one to

**Figure 4.3  The Plan-Do-Study-Act (PSDA) Cycle for Learning and Improvement**

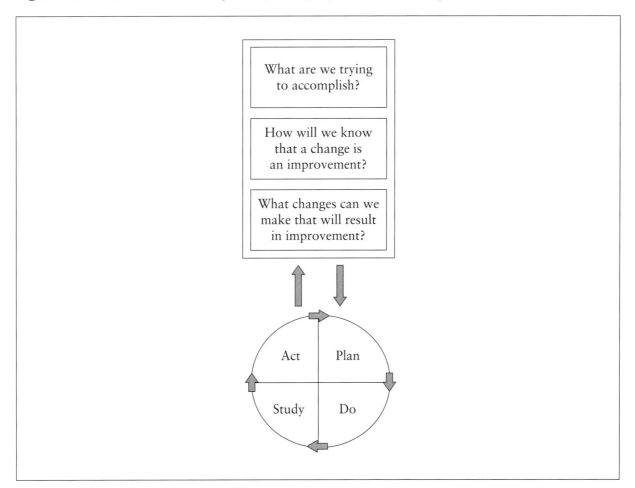

Source: Institute for Healthcare Improvement. Science of Improvement: How to Improve. http://www.ihi.org/resources/
Pages/HowtoImprove/ScienceofImprovementHowtoImprove.aspx. Last accessed March 23, 2015.

test changes in the real-world work environment. It is used to assess if changes will really make an improvement. The PDSA cycle is not meant to replace change models, but to assist in accelerating improvement and allows for testing change on a smaller scale.

Key Points:

- Keep the project small. In Case 5, the CQI team worked with one provider and the provider's patient panel. The provider's patient panel represented approximately 50 patients that fit the above criteria.
- Create a tracking sheet that tracks your outcomes. You don't need a lot of data to identify your problem; just make sure you are tracking the important data.
- Share your findings with the rest of the CQI team members and beyond. Help your team understand why this is a problem and brainstorm how to fix it.
- Remember, CQI and PDSA are cycles of improvement—once you have identified a way to act, complete a new cycle and track your outcomes.

# Appendix I   The CQI Process and the Research Process

The CQI process may generate research questions that can be generalized to improve diabetes education programs and patient health outcomes. It is important for diabetes educators to understand the relationship between CQI and research. Confusion about the distinction between CQI and research sometimes leads to the misconception that the processes are interchangeable. A 2007 article in the *Annals of Internal Medicine* contrasted QI with research activities, noting that QI[55]:

- is designed to bring about immediate improvements in healthcare delivery
- is designed to have its findings applicable only to the local institution
- is designed to sustain the improvements
- does not require rigid, fixed protocols; within QI activities it is acceptable to adapt the project over time

Table 5.1 provides a side-by-side comparison of the characteristics of CQI and research.

**Table 5.1   Comparison of CQI and Research**

| Characteristic | CQI | Research |
|---|---|---|
| Purpose | Improve a local process to benefit patients and providers; required by institution, regulatory, or accrediting agencies | Discover knowledge to benefit a larger population |
| Approach | Retrospective or concurrent | Laboratory and clinical research |
| Institutional Review Board (IRB) approval | Sometimes required | Required |
| Data source | Usually chart review | Various sources such as lab data, observational data |
| Sample size | Usually 5% to 10% of the population to be studied | Sufficient to provide statistical power |
| Performed by | Clinicians and managers who are part of the process being studied | People who are not part of the process |
| Time frame | Continuous or cyclical | Fixed endpoint |
| Communication of results | Within the institution | Outside the institution |

Source: Adapted from Marchette L, Holloman F. The research-quality assessment connection. *Journal of Healthcare Quality.* 2003;25(4):41.

The differences between the two processes must be understood before one can examine the similarities. The steps for CQI and research are compared in Table 5.2.

There is a fine line between CQI and research. Your CQI project may be adaptable to a larger population outside of your immediate practice setting and may have the potential to improve diabetes outcomes and health care for more patients. Such a benefit can only be identified and measured through research.

**Table 5.2  Steps for CQI and Research**

| Step | CQI | Research |
|:---:|---|---|
| 1 | Identify problem/opportunity | Identify a problem |
| 2 | Collect data:<br>• Define sample<br>• Choose data collection method<br>• Choose or develop data collection tools | Choose approach:<br>• Retrospective or Prospective<br>• Descriptive<br>• Correlational<br>• Experimental |
| 3 | Analyze data and draw conclusions | Conduct literature review |
| 4 | Identify alternative solutions | State purpose/hypotheses |
| 5 | Develop implementation plan and communicate findings | Choose evaluation instrument |
| 6 | Implement the plan | Define sample |
| 7 | Evaluate actions | Choose data collection method |
| 8 | Maintain improvement | • Write proposal and obtain approval for study<br>• Conduct pilot study<br>• Obtain funding<br>• Select sample<br>• Collect data<br>• Organize/analyze data<br>• Draw conclusions<br>• Make recommendations<br>• Write report<br>• Communicate findings |

Source: Adapted from Marchette L, Holloman F. The research-quality assessment connection. *Journal of Healthcare Quality.* 2003;25(4):41.

# Appendix II   Analytic Tools and Methods

There are numerous methods for displaying data that you've collected as part of your CQI process. This appendix lists some of the more common tools, describes the best use of the tool, and offers some cautions when using the tool. Depending on the size and focus of your CQI project, your CQI team should either include data experts or be sure to consult data experts at your institution to select the methods and tools that are best suited for your CQI project.

## Flowchart

A flowchart is a graphical method for displaying a sequence of steps, activities, or decision points that occur in a specific process or an algorithm. A flowchart helps to clarify how things are working currently and how things could be improved. It also assists in finding the key elements of a process, while drawing clear lines between where one process ends and the next one starts. In a healthcare setting, flowcharts can be used to examine processes for the flow of patients, information, materials, clinical care, or combinations of these processes. Flowcharts are best developed through group discussion, as individuals rarely know the entire process.

Use flowcharts to

- understand processes
- consider ways to simplify processes
- recognize unnecessary steps in a process
- determine areas for monitoring or data collection
- identify who will be involved in or affected by the improvement process
- formulate questions for further research

There are several types of flowcharts: high-level, detailed, and deployment or matrix.

### High-Level Flowchart

A high-level flowchart (also called *first-level* or *top-down flowchart*) depicts the major steps in a process. It illustrates a bird's-eye view of a process. It can also include the intermediate outputs of each step (the product or service produced) and the sub-steps involved. This type of flowchart offers a basic picture of the process and identifies the changes taking place within the process.

Use a high-level flowchart to

- identify individuals involved in the process
- develop indicators for monitoring the process

### Detailed Flowchart

A detailed flowchart indicates all the steps or activities of a process and includes such things as decision points, waiting periods, tasks that frequently must be redone, and feedback loops.

Use a detailed flowchart to

- examine areas of the process in detail
- look for problems or areas of inefficiency

## Deployment or Matrix Flowchart

A deployment flowchart maps out the process in terms of who is doing the steps. It is in the form of a matrix, which shows the various participants and the flow of steps among these participants.

Use a deployment or matrix flowchart to

- identify who is providing inputs or services to whom
- identify areas where different individuals may be needlessly doing the same task

## Tips for Using Flowcharts

- Be sure the flowchart focuses only on the identified problem and does not include irrelevant information.
- If ideas for improvement are generated during the flowchart development process, note them for a separate discussion. Do not discuss the merit of these ideas or include them in the flowchart.
- Be sure the steps and decision points your CQI team puts in the flowchart reflect the processes as they are being done currently and *not* how they should be done.
- Involve the individuals who know the process as part of the team developing the flowchart or as reviewers of the completed chart.

# Cause-and-Effect Analysis

A cause-and-effect analysis generates and sorts hypotheses about causes of problems within a process by asking participants to list all of the possible causes and effects of the identified problem. This analysis tool organizes a large amount of information by showing links between events and their potential or actual causes. It provides a method for generating ideas about why the problem is occurring and possible effects of that cause. Cause-and-effect analyses allow your CQI team to broaden its thinking and look at the overall picture of a problem. Cause-and-effect diagrams can reflect either causes that block the way to the desired state or helpful factors needed to reach the desired state.

There are two ways to graphically organize ideas for a cause-and-effect analysis:

1. Category—a *fishbone diagram* (for its shape) or *Ishikawa diagram* (for the man who invented it)
2. A chain of causes—a *tree diagram*

## Causes by Category (Fishbone Diagram)

The fishbone diagram helps your CQI team to brainstorm about possible causes of a problem, accumulate existing knowledge about the causal system surrounding that problem, and group causes into general categories. (See Figure 3.2.)

Use a fishbone diagram to display categories of causation:

- Human resources, methods, materials, measurements, and equipment
- Clients, workers, supplies, environment, and procedures
- What, how, when, where

## Chain of Causes (Tree Diagram)

The tree diagram highlights the sequence of the causes. The tree diagram is a graphical display of another method called the *Five Whys*. This graphic displays the layers of causes and is focused on finding the root cause.

Use a tree diagram to answer the following questions:

- Why is this happening?
- What is causing this?

# Bar and Pie Charts

Bar and pie charts use pictures to compare the sizes, amounts, quantities, or proportions of various items or groupings of items. They can be used in defining or choosing problems to work on, analyzing problems, verifying causes, or judging solutions. Bar charts work best when showing comparisons among categories. Pie charts work well for presenting relative proportions of various items that make up the whole, i.e., how the "pie" is divided.

There are several types of bar charts. The choice of bar chart should be based on the type of data that your CQI team has and what points about the data that the team wants to highlight.

- *Simple bar charts* sort data into simple categories.
- *Grouped bar charts* divide data into groups within each category and show comparisons between individual groups as well as between categories. This type of bar chart provides more useful information than a simple total of all the components.
- *Stacked bar charts* also use grouped data within categories. This type of chart clearly displays the sum of the parts as well as each group's contribution to that total.

Use bar charts and pie charts to

- define or choose problems to work on
- analyze problems
- verify causes
- judge solutions

### Tips for Using Bar and Pie Charts

- Scales must be in regular intervals.
- Charts that are to be compared must have the same scale and symbols.
- Charts should be easy to read.
- Keep the charts as simple as possible. Include only the information necessary to interpret the chart. Be careful not to use too many notations on the charts.
- Keep in mind that bar and pie charts are not intended to convey complicated data well. Don't draw conclusions that the data can't justify. For example, trends and differences among groups may require more statistical testing and analysis and probably can't be determined by the chart alone.

## Run Chart

Run charts provide graphical presentation of a variation in some process over time and help detect special (external) causes of that variation. They make trends or other nonrandom variation in the process easier to see and understand. With the understanding of patterns and trends of the past, groups can then use run charts to help predict future performance.

Use a run chart to

- detect trends over time
- determine if there is a change in a process
- monitor progress of solutions

### Tips for Using Run Charts

- Scales must be in regular intervals.
- Charts that are to be compared must have the same scale and symbols.
- Charts should be easy to read.
- Keep the charts as simple as possible. Include only the information necessary to interpret the chart. Be careful not to use too many notations on the charts.
- Do not draw conclusions that the data can't justify. Certain trends and interpretations may require more statistical testing to determine if they are significant.

## Histogram

A histogram is a graphical display of a single variable in a bar form to indicate how often some event is likely to occur by showing the pattern of variation (distribution) of data. A pattern of variation has three aspects: the center (average), the shape of the curve, and the width of the curve. Histograms are constructed with variables—such as time, weight, temperature—and are not appropriate for attribute data.

There are several types of histograms:

- *Bell shaped:* The normal pattern
- *Double peaked:* Suggests two distributions
- *Skewed:* Look for other processes in the tail
- *Truncated:* Look for reasons for sharp end of distribution or pattern
- *Ragged plateau:* No single clear process or pattern

Use a histogram to

- identify and verify causes of problems
- judge a solution, by checking whether it has removed the cause of the problem

## Tips for Using Histograms

If variation is small, the histogram may not be sensitive enough to detect significant differences in variability or in the peaks of the distribution, especially if using a small-sample data set. There are advanced statistical tools that can be used in such situations.

# Scatter Diagrams

The scatter diagram is a graphical visual display of data that shows the association between two variables acting continuously on the same item. (Continuous data are things like time, numbers, and temperature.) The scatter diagram illustrates the strength of the *correlation* between the variables through the slope of a line. This correlation can point to, but does not prove, a *causal* relationship. The scatter diagram is easy to use, but should be interpreted with caution as the scale may be too small to see the relationship between variables, or confounding factors may be involved.

Use a scatter diagram to

- help determine if there is a relationship between two variables
- quickly test the relationship between two variables

## Tips for Using Scatter Diagrams

- Stratifying the data in different ways can make patterns appear or disappear. When experimenting with different stratifications and their effects on the scatter diagram, label how the data are stratified so the team can discuss the implications.
- Interpretation can be limited by the scale used. If the scale is too small and the points are compressed, then a pattern of correlation may appear differently. Determine the scale so that the points cover most of the range of both axes and that both axes are about the same length.
- Be careful of the effects of confounding factors. Sometimes the correlation observed is due to some cause other than the one being studied. If a confounding factor is suspected, then stratify the data by it. If it is truly a confounding factor, then the relationship in the diagram will change significantly.

- Avoid the temptation to draw a line roughly through the middle of the points. This can be misleading. A true regression line is determined mathematically. Consult a statistical expert or text prior to using a regression line.
- Scatter diagrams show relationships but do not prove that one variable causes the other.

# Pareto Chart

A Pareto chart organizes and displays information to show the relative importance of various problems or causes of problems. It is essentially a special form of a vertical bar chart that puts items in order, from the highest to the lowest, relative to some measurable effect of interest: frequency, cost, time.

Pareto charts help your CQI team focus on the small number of important problems or causes of problems. Pareto charts are useful in establishing priorities by showing which are the most critical problems to be tackled or causes to be addressed. By comparing Pareto charts of a specific situation over time, your CQI team can also determine whether an implemented solution reduced the relative frequency or cost of that problem or cause.

Use Pareto charts to

- focus on areas of priority
- quickly organize priorities in a graphical format

# Benchmarking

Best practices benchmarking is a systematic approach for gathering information about process or product performance and analyzing why and how performance differs between entities or departments within the same organization. Benchmarking is a technique for learning from the success of others in an area where your CQI team is trying to make improvements. Sources of information for benchmarking include literature reviews, databases, unions, standard-setting organizations, local organizations, universities, the government, staff or customer interviews, and questionnaires.

Use benchmarking to

- develop options for potential solutions
- borrow and adapt successful ideas from others
- understand what has already been tried and what has been successful

### Tips for Using Benchmarking

- Before looking at others' processes, be sure your CQI team completely understands how the process works in your setting.
- Be sure that the other facility's process is fully understood before adapting or adopting it to the process your CQI team is addressing.

# Gantt Chart

A Gantt chart aids planning by showing all activities that must take place and when they are scheduled to occur. This tool helps your CQI team visualize the work that needs to be completed, the activities that can be overlapped, and deadlines for completion. Gantt charts are most useful in the planning stages, to mark when each activity should start and to draw the linkages in timing between activities. Gantt charts are also useful for keeping track of progress and rescheduling activities if progress is slowed.

Use Gantt charts to

- plan quality improvement projects according to activities and time
- understand the overlap and sequence of activities
- monitor progress and reevaluate deadlines if the project is behind schedule

# Quality Assurance Storytelling

Quality assurance storytelling is an organized way of documenting the quality improvement process of your CQI team. Initially developed as quality improvement storytelling for industrial programs, the technique has more recently been adapted and applied to quality improvement efforts in the healthcare sector. The quality assurance (QA) stories or narratives are described in detail in QA *storybook*s and presented publicly through QA *storyboard*s.

The QA storybook is a complete and permanent record of the improvement process, which is usually kept in notebook format, though there are creative methods for producing this online, too. The QA storyboard is a large display area (e.g., section of a wall, or a board or poster) that allows your CQI team to display its work publicly in an ongoing, structured, and visually understandable way.

Use quality assurance storytelling to

- systematically document the quality improvement process of your CQI team
- help make the CQI/QA process part of the ongoing life of your organization

# Appendix III  Application to Your Practice Worksheets

## Worksheet 1.1  Understanding Your Customers

| | |
|---|---|
| **Identify Your Customers** | |
| Who are your most important *internal* customers? | |
| Who are the decision makers and/or individuals within your organization that can have an impact on your DSME program? | |
| Who are your most important *external* customers? | |
| Who are the individuals and/or organizations that can have an impact on your DSME program? | |
| **Identify Your Customers' Needs** | |
| What do your *internal* customers want from your DSME program? | |
| What do your *external* customers want from your DSME program? | |
| **Ask for Customer Feedback** | |
| How do you think your *internal* customers would rate the efficiency and effectiveness of your DSME program? | |
| Survey your *internal* customers to see if their responses match your assumptions. | |
| How do you think your *external* customers would rate the efficiency and effectiveness of your DSME program? | |
| Survey your *external* customers to see if their responses match your assumptions. | |
| **Fill In the Gaps** | |
| What information do you lack about your *internal* customers? | |
| What information do you lack about your *external* customers? | |

## Worksheet 3.1  CQI Team Candidates

Assess proposed team candidate on each of the team role indicators.

**Candidate Name:** _____  **Role on Team:** _____

| Team Role Indicators | Yes | No | Possibly | Comments |
|---|---|---|---|---|
| Demonstrates a clear understanding and support of the project goals and objectives. | | | | |
| Is able to commit the time and attention required for role on the project team. | | | | |
| Possesses the collaboration and communication skills appropriate to the project role. | | | | |
| Possesses the skills and knowledge required for role on the project team. | | | | |
| **Identify the specific strengths and weaknesses this candidate brings to the role on the team** | | | | |
| Skills/knowledge that may positively affect performance in role on the team. | | | | |
| Skill/knowledge gaps or deficiencies that may negatively affect performance on the team. | | | | |

## Worksheet 3.2  Project Reporting Form

| Project Title | | | | | |
|---|---|---|---|---|---|
| Project Team Members | Last Name | First Name | Role on Team | E-mail | Phone |
| | | | | | |
| | | | | | |
| | | | | | |
| | | | | | |

| Date | Agenda/Topics | Notes | Action(s) Required | Responsible Team Member(s) |
|---|---|---|---|---|
| | | | | |
| | | | | |
| | | | | |
| | | | | |
| | | | | |
| | | | | |
| | | | | |
| | | | | |
| | | | | |
| | | | | |
| | | | | |

## Worksheet 3.3 Potential CQI Projects

1. Column A: Identify areas for improvement within your diabetes education program. At this time, do not evaluate the potential of the suggestion as a CQI project. Do not try to identify solutions.

2. Column B: Write a desired outcome to address each item identified in Column A.

   Use the information collected in this form to help you determine which problem identified in Column A has the best potential as a successful project outcome.

| A | B |
|---|---|
| **Problems/Areas for Improvement** | **Desired Outcome** |
|  |  |
|  |  |
|  |  |
|  |  |
|  |  |
|  |  |

**Worksheet 3.4   Data Collection for Your CQI Project**

| | |
|---|---|
| What data do you need for your CQI project? | |
| Who owns or manages the data? | |
| In what format(s) are the data available, e.g., database, paper files, electronic files? What are the file format(s) of the electronic files? What database program is being used? | |
| Will the CQI team members require training to collect and analyze the data? | |
| Are these data available to you in a format that is usable for your project? | |
| How will the data be collected? | |
| Is there a cost to collect the data? Do you need to purchase or have access to specific software to collect and work with the data? | |
| Who will be involved in the data collection, e.g., both CQI team members and individuals/departments that own the data? | |
| What is the contact information for everyone involved in the data collection? | |

## Worksheet 3.5   The CQI Process and Its Applications to Your Practice

Reflect on what you have learned about the CQI process and its applications to your day-to-day practice.

| | |
|---|---|
| What steps in your CQI project worked well? | |
| What steps in your CQI project could be improved? | |
| Evaluate your team performance. What changes would you make to the team selection process, training, assignments, other? | |
| Identify resources that you would want in place for your next CQI project. | |
| Did the CQI project deliver the expected outcome(s)? Why/why not? If not, can you identify areas in the process that may have contributed? | |
| Did the CQI process deliver unanticipated outcomes—positive or negative? Can you identify areas in the process that may have contributed to these unanticipated outcomes? | |

# Glossary

**ACA**

See *Patient Protection and Affordable Care Act (PPACA)*.

**ACO**

See *Accountable Care Organizations (ACOs)*.

**Accountable Care Organizations (ACOs)**

A network of doctors, hospitals, and other healthcare providers that share responsibility for providing care to patients. The ACO is characterized by a payment and care delivery model that seeks to tie provider reimbursements to quality metrics and reductions in the total cost of care for an assigned population of patients. The ACO is accountable to the patients and the third-party payers for the quality, appropriateness, and efficiency of the health care provided. Section 3022 of the Patient Protection and Affordable Care Act (ACA) authorizes the Centers for Medicare and Medicaid Services (CMS) to create the Medicare Shared Savings program (MSSP), which allows for the establishment of ACO contracts with Medicare.

**Accreditation**

A formal process in which an official or independent review agency acknowledges that the institution or individual seeking accreditation meets predetermined standard(s) of practice; required for third-party reimbursement.

**Affinity Diagram**

A tool used to collect large amounts of language data, e.g., ideas, issues, or opinions, from brainstorming sessions. The data are grouped together based on their relationship with one another. For example, ideas for CQI projects might be grouped under the headings of behavioral, clinical, and program.

**Aggregate-Level Outcomes**

Pooled data that are routinely assessed, summarized, and reported.

**Algorithm**

A mathematical rule or procedure for solving a problem.

**Bar Chart**

A graphical method for displaying data in the form of a stripe(s) or a bar(s) that shows the number of units (e.g., frequency) in each category.

**Baseline**

Data that serve as the starting point for comparisons with subsequently collected data.

**Benchmark**

A standard or measurement or evaluation. Benchmarks may be *internal* (established within the organization, *external* (from an outside organization that produces the same service or product), or *functional* (from an outside organization in a different industry, but referencing a similar function or process).

**Benchmarking**

A process of researching and assessing the best practices that produce superior performance.

**Best Practices**

A way or method of accomplishing a function or process that is considered to be superior to other known functions or processes.

**Bias**

A systematic error introduced through some aspect of the study design.

**Brainstorming**

A group problem-solving method in which all members of the group generate ideas spontaneously and without judgment or assessment of the ideas.

**CCM**

See *Chronic Care Model.*

**CQI**

See *Continuous Quality Improvement.*

**Case-Control Study**

An observational study which begins with the identification of a group of cases (individuals with the condition of interest) and a group of suitable controls (individuals without the condition). The level of exposure to a risk factor is measured in the two groups and compared.

**Cause-and-Effect Diagram**

See *Fishbone Diagram.*

**Check Sheet/Checklist**

Usually a blank form with columns or rows labeled with information that needs to be tracked. A check sheet can be used to record qualitative or quantitative information.

## Chronic Care Model (CCM)

A model for evidence-based healthcare system changes that meet the needs of growing numbers of people who have chronic disease. CCM was developed to provide patients with self-management skills and tracking systems. The model represents an approach to restructuring medical care through partnerships between health systems and communities.

## Clinical Practice Guidelines

Set of systematically developed statements generally based on scientific evidence that practitioners use when making decisions about appropriate healthcare choices for a specific clinical circumstance.

## Clinical Research

Type of research that involves direct observation and treatment of patients.

## Cohort Study

A study in which a group of individuals who were exposed to a potential risk and a group of individuals who were not exposed to a potential risk factor are studied for a length of time after the exposure/lack of exposure to the risk factor. The incidence of the outcome in one group is compared with the incidence in the other. Also called a *follow-up study* or a *longitudinal study*.

## Concurrent Data Collection

Method of collecting current data while a study is being conducted, from baseline exam to end of study.

## Confidence Interval

Describes the uncertainty associated with a *sampling method*.

## Confounding

Occurs when there is a mixing of the effects between the exposure and the outcome being studied and a third factor that is associated with the exposure, but can independently affect the risk of the outcome.

## Continuous Quality Improvement (CQI)

Process that consists of a series of steps designed to enhance DSME and improve patient and program outcomes; steps include identifying the opportunity for improvement, collecting data, analyzing data, choosing an approach, developing concepts and processes, implementing a plan, evaluating the plan, and maintaining the improvement.

## Control Chart

A graphical method used to display the results of a process over time and against established control limits. Control charts are used to determine whether a process is in a state of statistical control. Also known as a *Shewhart chart* or a *process-behavior chart*.

## Correlational Study

Explores the statistical connection between disease in different population groups and estimated exposures in groups rather than individuals.

## Cross-Sectional Study

A study in which information on the risk factors and the outcomes are measured simultaneously at one point in time.

## EHR

See *Electronic Medical Record (EMR)*.

## EMR

See *Electronic Medical Record (EMR)*.

## Ecologic Study

A study in which the units of analysis are populations or groups of people rather than individuals. Also called an *aggregate risk study*.

## Electronic Health Record (EHR)

See *Electronic Medical Record (EMR)*.

## Electronic Medical Record (EMR)

Also called an **electronic health record (EHR)**. A systematic collection of electronic health information about an individual patient or population designed to represent data that accurately capture the state of the patient at all times. It allows for an entire patient history to be viewed without the need to track down the patient's previous medical record volume and assists in ensuring data are accurate, appropriate, and legible. It is a record in digital format that is theoretically capable of being shared across different healthcare settings. In some cases this sharing can occur by way of network-connected, enterprise-wide information systems and other information networks or exchanges. EMRs may include a range of data, such as demographics, medical history, medication and allergies, immunization status, laboratory test results, radiology images, vital signs, personal statistics like age and weight, and billing information.

## Evaluation

The act of examining processes and outcomes to determine whether the desired goals and objectives (individual or program) were achieved.

## Evidence-Based Medicine

Practices, procedures, and interventions that are guided by or based on supportive scientific evidence. Evidence-based also means the avoidance of those interventions shown by scientific evidence to be harmful or ineffective.

**Experimental Study**

A study in which the conditions are under the direct control of the investigator.

**Fishbone Diagram**

A graphical method for displaying the many possible causes of a problem. This diagram's name is a result of its resemblance to the skeleton of a fish. The problem is represented by the main line (or spine), while the possible causes are represented by lines (or bones) drawn vertically from the main line. Also known as a *cause-and-effect diagram* and the *Ishikawa diagram*, after its inventor, Dr. Kaoru Ishikawa.

**Flowchart**

A graphical method for displaying a sequence of steps, activities, or decision points that occur in a specific process or an algorithm.

**Gantt Chart**

A type of bar chart used in process or project planning and control. Displays planned work targets for completion of tasks in relation to time, e.g., the chart shows the month in which the task will be completed and the individual(s) responsible for each task.

**HIPAA**

See *Health Insurance Portability and Accountability Act (HIPAA)*.

**Health Insurance Portability and Accountability Act (HIPAA)**

Officially known as the United States Health Insurance Portability and Accountability Act of 1996. There are two sections to the Act. HIPAA Title I addresses the protection of health insurance coverage for individuals who lose their job or who change jobs. Title II addresses, among other things, the standardization of healthcare-related information systems. HIPAA mandates standardized formats for all patient health, administrative, and financial data; unique identifiers (ID numbers) for each healthcare entity, including individuals, employers, health plans, and healthcare providers; and security mechanisms to ensure confidentiality and data integrity for any information that identifies an individual.

**Health Outcomes**

End results of a health-related study; typically reflect the measurement of learning and behavioral, clinical, and functional status, as well as patient-centered outcomes of satisfaction and well-being.

**Histogram**

A graphical display of tabulated frequencies. A histogram shows what proportion of cases fall into each of the specified categories.

**IRB**

See *Institutional Review Board (IRB)*.

### Immediate Outcomes

Can be measured at the time of the intervention, e.g., learning as assessed by testing or direct observation.

### Indicator

A measurable variable or characteristic that can be used to determine the degree of adherence to a standard or the level of quality achieved.

### Institutional Review Board (IRB)

A committee that oversees patient safety and the scientific merit of research projects that are conducted at the practice setting where this group has jurisdiction.

### Intermediate and Post-Intermediate Outcomes

Outcomes that result over time, require more than a single measurement, are sensitive to change, and may show a statistical change, e.g., behavior change or clinical improvements.

### Long-Term Outcomes

Result from multiple variables over an extended time, e.g., improve health or quality of life.

### Margin of Error

The margin of error expresses the maximum expected difference between the true population parameter and a sample estimate of that parameter. To be meaningful, the margin of error should be qualified by a probability statement (often expressed in the form of a confidence level).

### Measure

A number assigned to an object or an event. Measures can be expressed in several different ways: counts (20 visits), rates (20 visits/day), proportions (20 primary healthcare visits/400 total visits = .050), percentage (5 percent of the visits made), or ratios (20 visits/4 health workers = 5).

### Measurement

Evaluation of a health outcomes indicator.

### Observational Study

A study in which the role of the investigator is to be an observer of what happens. Examples of observational studies include case-control, cohort, and cross-sectional studies. Also called *non-experimental study*.

### Outcomes

End results of the delivery of healthcare services or a research study.

**Outcomes Management**

Application of data from outcomes measurement and monitoring that are used to guide decision making regarding the delivery of an intervention or service.

**Outcomes Measurement**

Assessment of indicators of health status, satisfaction, survival, and costs as associated with the delivery of healthcare services.

**Outcomes Monitoring**

Process of measuring the frequency and interval of outcomes.

**PCMH**

See *Patient-Centered Medical Home (PCMH)*.

**Pareto Chart**

A type of bar chart that ranks the categories by frequency, cost, time, or money. The tallest bars are placed on the left in the chart and the shortest on the right. Originally developed by Vilfredo Pareto for use in analyzing economic data.

**Patient Protection and Affordable Care Act (ACA)**

Also known as the *Affordable Care Act (ACA)* or *Obamacare*. Signed into law in March of 2010, with provisions and rolled out between 2010 and 2014. Key provisions are intended to extend coverage to millions of uninsured Americans, to implement measures that will lower healthcare costs and improve system efficiency, and to eliminate industry practices that include rescission and denial of coverage due to preexisting conditions.

**Patient-Centered Medical Home (PCMH)**

A model that organizes primary health care to emphasize care coordination and communication. Designed to lead to higher-quality care, lower costs, and improvement in the patients' and providers' experience of care.

**Performance Measurement**

Objective evaluation and quantification of a healthcare indicator, such as quality; the first step in the process of performance measurement, assessment, and improvement; similar to the outcomes measurement process that involves measurement, monitoring, and management.

**Post-Immediate Outcomes**

See *Intermediate Outcomes*.

**Problem Solving**

A quality improvement approach that involves objectively identifying the causes of a problem and proposing potential solutions.

## Problem Statement

A concise description of a process that is in need of improvement. The statement includes the scope, focus, and limits of the work, as well as an explanation of why work on the improvement is a priority.

## Process

A series of actions (or activities) that transforms inputs (or resources) into a desired product, service, or outcome.

## Process Measures

Procedures that describe what a healthcare service provides or delivers.

## Program Evaluation

The systematic collection of information about the activities, characteristics, and outcomes of programs to make judgments about the program, improve program effectiveness, and/or inform decisions about future program development.

## Prospective Data Collection

A method of collecting data over a period of time to learn what factor(s) may be causing a particular problem or characteristic.

## Protocol

A detailed plan or a set of steps to be followed in a study, an investigation, or an intervention.

## Quality Assurance

An indication of the level of adherence to quality indicators and healthcare standards.

## Quality Improvement

A continuous process that identifies problems in healthcare delivery, looks for solutions to those problems/solutions for improvement, and regularly monitors the solutions to those problems/solutions for improvement.

## Quality Indicator

A measurable variable or characteristic that can be used to determine the degree of adherence to a standard or achievement of quality goals.

## Rate

A proportion that includes specification of time, e.g., the amputation rate of people diagnosed with Type I diabetes is the number of cases of people diagnosed with Type I diabetes who underwent an amputation within a defined time period divided by the total number of cases of people diagnosed with Type I diabetes in the same time period.

## Ratio

The relationship between two numbers, e.g., fractions, percentages, proportions, or quotients.

## Retrospective Data Collection

A method of collecting historical data from archives or records, e.g., medical chart provides information on outcomes that have already occurred.

## Run Chart

A graphical display of data over time that indicates how well/badly a process is being performed and whether or not a change in process results in a change in outcomes.

## Sample

A subset of the population being studied. Ideally, the sample should be as representative as possible of the larger population from which it is drawn.

## Sample Size

The number of individuals or objectives being studied.

## Scatter Diagram

A graphical display where the data are represented as a collection of points. Each point is the value of one variable, which determines its position on the horizontal and vertical axes.

## Standard

A statement that defines expectations of quality within a particular area, which, if adhered to, should help meet the highest possible level of quality within that area.

## Standard Deviation

A numerical value used to indicate how widely individuals in a group vary. If individual observations vary greatly from the group mean, the standard deviation is big, and vice versa. The standard deviation of a population and a sample are computed differently and have different notations.

## Threshold

A level of achievement that determines the difference between what is deemed to be acceptable quality and what is not. For example, "the minimal acceptable level of coverage for the immunization program is 50 percent" means that every coverage figure less than that is an indication of a quality problem.

## Time Series Graph

A graphical display in the form of a line graph in which time is measured on the horizontal axis and the variable being observed is measured on the vertical axis.

## Time Study

An analysis of a specific job, task, or process done in an effort to determine the most efficient method in terms of time and effort.

## Validity

The degree to which an indicator accurately measures what it is intended to measure.

## Variation

The differences in the output of a process that can result from the influence of a variety of things, such as equipment, individuals, materials, or methods.

# References

1. National diabetes fact sheet: national estimates and general information on diabetes and prediabetes in the United States, 2011. Atlanta, GA: U.S. Department of Health and Human Services, Centers for Disease Control and Prevention; 2011.

2. American Diabetes Association. Economic costs of diabetes in the U.S. in 2012. *Diabetes Care.* 2013;36(4):1033-1046.

3. Institute for Healthcare Improvement (IHI). Triple Aim. http://www.ihi.org/engage/initiatives/TripleAim/Pages/default.aspx. Last accessed 03.23.15.

4. Mosby's Medical Dictionary, 8th edition. © 2009, Elsevier. Mosby's Dictionary of Medicine, Nursing & Health Professions, 2012.

5. Going Lean in Health Care. IHI Innovation Series white paper. Cambridge, MA: Institute for Healthcare Improvement; 2005.

6. Kemp S. Quality Management Demystified. New York: McGraw-Hill Professional; 2005:21-39.

7. Ibid., 177-190.

8. Ibid., 191-204.

9. University Alliance. Six Sigma vs. Lean Six Sigma. http://www.villanovau.com/resources/six-sigma/six-sigma-vs-lean-six-sigma/#.VQCy6Xoo6Uk. Last accessed 03.23.15.

10. Six Sigma Online. Lean Six Sigma vs. Traditional Six Sigma. http://www.sixsigmaonline.org/six-sigma-training-certification-information/articles/lean-six-sigma-vs-traditional-six-sigma.html. Last accessed 03.23.15.

11. Kemp S. Quality Management Demystified. New York: McGraw-Hill Professional; 2005: 247-262.

12. Patient Protection and Affordable Care Act, 42 U.S.C. § 18001 (2010).

13. Centers for Medicare and Medicaid Services. Accountable Care Organizations. http://www.cms.gov/Medicare/Medicare-Fee-for-Service-Payment/ACO/index.html?redirect=/ACO. Last accessed 03.23.15.

14. National Committee on Quality Assurance. HEDIS & Performance Measurement. http://www.ncqa.org/HEDISQualityMeasurement.aspx. Last accessed 03.23.15.

15. American College of Physicians. CME Credit and MOC Points for Patient Safety Module. http://www.acponline.org/education_recertification/recertification/resources/patient_safety_moc/. Last accessed 03.23.15.

16. American Board of Internal Medicine. ABIM MOC—Helping Physicians Improve Quality of Care. September 2012. http://www.scribd.com/doc/111478081/ABIM-MOC-Helping-Physicians-IMPROVE-QUALITY-CARE#scribd. Last accessed 03.23.15.

17. Department of Health and Human Services. Administration on Aging—Aging Statistics. http://www.aoa.gov/Aging_Statistics/. Last accessed 03.23.15.

18. Centers for Disease Control and Prevention. Chronic Disease Prevention and Health Promotion—Chronic Diseases and Health Promotion. http://www.cdc.gov/chronicdisease/overview/. Last accessed 03.23.15.

19. Committee on Quality of Health Care in America, Institute of Medicine. Crossing the Quality Chasm: A New Health System for the 21st Century. Washington, D.C.: National Academies Press; 2001.

20. Committee on Redesigning Health Insurance Performance Measures, Payment, and Performance Improvement Programs, Institute of Medicine. Performance Measurement: Accelerating Improvement (Pathways to Quality Health Care Series). Washington, D.C.: National Academy Press; 2006.

21. Dentzer S. Still crossing the quality chasm—or suspended over it? *Health Aff.* 2011;30(4):554-555.

22. Wagner EH, Austin BT, Davis C, Hindmarsh M, Schaefer J, Bonomi A. Improving chronic illness care: translating evidence into action. *Health Aff.* (Millwood). 2001;20:64-78.

23. Improving Chronic Illness Care. Regional Framework: Introduction. http://www.improving chroniccare.org/index.php?p=Regional_Framework&s=50. Last accessed 03.23.15.

24. California Healthcare Foundation. It Takes a Region: Creating a Framework to Improve Chronic Disease Care. November 2006. http://www.chcf.org/~/media/MEDIA%20LIBRARY%20Files/PDF/C/PDF%20CreatingAFrameworkToImproveChronicDiseaseCare.pdf. Last accessed 03.23.15.

25. Robert Wood Johnson Foundation. Improving the Science of Continuous Quality Improvement Program and Evaluation. June 25, 2012. http://www.rwjf.org/content/dam/farm/reports/program_results_reports/2012/rwjf73230. Last accessed 03.23.15.

26. Agency for Healthcare Research and Quality. A Decade of Evidence, Design, and Implementation: Advancing Patient Safety. September 2012. http://www.ahrq.gov/professionals/quality-patient-safety/patient-safety-resources/resources/advancing-patient-safety/index.html. Last accessed 03.23.15.

27. Patient-Centered Primary Care Collaborative (PCPCC). Joint Principles of the Patient-Centered Medical Home. http://www.aafp.org/dam/AAFP/documents/practice_management/pcmh/initia tives/PCMHJoint.pdf. Last accessed 03.23.15.

28. Patient-Centered Primary Care Collaborative (PCPCC). Defining the Medical Home. http://www.pcpcc.org/about/medical-home. Last accessed 03.23.15.

29. Gabbay RA, Friedberg MW, Miller-Day M, Cronholm PF, Adelman A, Schneider EC. A positive deviance approach to understanding key features to improving diabetes care in the medical home. *Ann Fam Med.* 2013;11(1):S99-S107.

30. Friedberg MW, Schneider EC, Rosenthal MB, Volpp KG, Werner RM. Association between participation in a multipayer medical home intervention and changes in quality, utilization, and costs of care. *JAMA.* 2014;311(8):815-25.

31. Higgins S, Chawla R, Colombo C, Snyder R, Nigam S. Medical homes and cost and utilization among high-risk patients. *AJMC.* 2014;20(3):e61-71.

32. Weaver C, Mathews A. An Rx? Pay more to family doctors. *Wall Street Journal.* Jan. 27, 2012.

33. Martin A, Hartman M, Whittle L, Catlin A, National Health Expenditure Accounts Team. National health spending in 2012: rate of health spending growth remain low for the fourth consecutive year. *Health Aff.* 2014;33(1):67-77.

34. Organisation for Economic Co-operation and Development (OECD). OECD Health Statistics 2014. http://www.oecd.org/health/health-systems/health-data.htm. Last accessed 03.23.15.

35. Berwick DM, Nolan TW, Whittington J. The Triple Aim: Care, health, and cost. *Health Aff.* 2008;27(3):759-769.

36. American Diabetes Association. Fast Facts Data and Statistics about Diabetes. http://professional.diabetes.org/ResourcesForProfessionals.aspx?cid=91777&loc=dorg-statistics. Last accessed 03.23.15.

37. Centers for Disease Control and Prevention. Number of Americans with Diabetes Projected to Double or Triple by 2050. http://www.cdc.gov/media/pressrel/2010/r101022.html. Last accessed 03.23.15.

38. American Diabetes Association. Economic costs of diabetes in the U.S. in 2012. *Diabetes Care.* 2013;36(4):1033-1046.

39. US Endocrinologist Shortage Affects Access to Care, Physician Satisfaction. *Endocrine Today.* May 2011.

40. Davidson JA. The increasing role of primary care physicians in caring for patients with type 2 diabetes mellitus. *Mayo Clin Proc.* 2010 Dec; 85(12 Suppl): S3-S4. doi: 10.4065/mcp.2010.0466 PMCID: PMC2996164

41. AADE7 Self-Care Behaviors Goal Sheet, part of AADE7™ System. Chicago, IL: American Association of Diabetes Educators (AADE). http://www.diabeteseducator.org. Last accessed 03.23.15.

42. Institute for Healthcare Improvement (IHI). Change Achievement Success Indicator (CASI). http://www.ihi.org/resources/Pages/Tools/ChangeAchievementSuccessIndicatorCASI.aspx. Last accessed 03.23.15.

43. Robert Wood Johnson Foundation. Tools for Continuous Quality Improvement. http://www.rwjf.org/en/how-we-work/rel/research-features/evaluating-CQI.html. Last accessed 03.23.15.

44. Institute for Healthcare Improvement (IHI). How to improve: Improvement methods. http://www.ihi.org/IHI/Topics/Improvement/ improvementmethods. Last accessed 03.23.15.

45. Hass L, Maryniuk M, Beck J., et al. National standards for diabetes self-management education and support. *Diabetes Educator.* 2012;38:619. doi: 10.1177/0145721712455997.

46. American Diabetes Association Recognition Programs. http://professional.diabetes.org/recognition.aspx. Last accessed 03.23.15.

47. American Association of Diabetes Educators Diabetes Education Accreditation Program (DEAP). www.diabeteseducator.org/ProfessionalResources/accred/. Last accessed 03.23.15.

48. Donabedian A. The Definition of Quality: A Conceptual Exploration. Ann Arbor, MI: Health Administration Press; 1980.

49. American Association of Diabetes Educators (AADE). AADE7 Self-Care Behaviors™. American Association of Diabetes Educators (AADE) Position Statement, December 3, 2014. http://

www.diabeteseducator.org/export/sites/aade/_resources/pdf/publications/AADE7_Position_Statement_Final.pdf. Last accessed 03.23.15.

50. Mulcahy K, Maryniuk M, Peeples M, et al. Diabetes self-management education core outcomes measures (technical review). *Diabetes Educ.* 2003;29(5):768-803.

51. American Health Care Association. CQI Climate Survey Report Generator. http://www.ahcancal.org. Last accessed 03.23.15.

52. Institute for Healthcare Improvement (IHI). http://www.ihi.org/IHI. Last accessed 03.23.15.

53. Mulcahy K. Management of diabetes education programs. In: Franz MJ, ed. A Core Curriculum for Diabetes Education and Program Management. 5th ed. Chicago, IL: American Association of Diabetes Educators; 2003:201.

54. Chapter 11, Quality improvement. In: Operations Manual for Delivery of HIV Prevention, Care and Treatment at Primary Health Centres in High-Prevalence, Resource-Constrained Settings. World Health Organization; 2008:295.

55. Grady C. Quality improvement and ethical oversight. *Ann Intern Med.* 2007;146(9):680-681.

# Index

Note: Page numbers of figures and tables are italicized.

## A

AADE7™ System
    Self-Care Behaviors Goal Sheet, 10, *17*, 21
Accountable care organizations (ACOs), 4–5
Affinity diagrams, *24*
Agency for Healthcare Research and Quality (AHRQ), 7
Alternative solutions, identifying, 31–32
American Association of Diabetes Educators (AADE)
    Diabetes Education Accreditation Program (DEAP), 12
American Board of Internal Medicine, 9
American Diabetes Association (ADA)
    Education Recognition Program (ERP), 12
American Health Care Association
    *CQI Climate Survey Report Generator*, 19
Analytic tools and methods, 51–57
    bar and pie charts, 53–54
    benchmarking, 13, *13*, *14–15*, 56
    cause-and-effect analysis, 52–53
    flowcharts, 51–52
    Gantt charts, 57
    histograms, 34–35, 54–55
    Pareto charts, 29–30, *30*, 56
    quality assurance storytelling, 57
    run charts, 28, 54
    scatter diagrams, 55–56
A1C measures, 16, 39–41, *40–42*
Attribute data, 25

## B

Bar charts, 53–54
Bell shaped histograms, 55
Benchmarking
    benefits of, *13*
    best practices, 56
    CQI measures, *14–15*
    definition of, 13

Berwick, Donald, 8–9
Brainstorming, 31

## C

Case studies, 39–47. *See also* CQI process
    evaluating behavior change in multiple sites, 45, *45–46*
    follow-up of high-risk patients, 46–47, *47*
    improving turnaround time, 44, *44*
    measuring behavior change, 42, *42*, *43*
    missing A1C data, 39–41, *40*, *41–42*
Categories of causation analysis. *See* Fishbone diagrams
Cause-and-effect analysis, 52–53
    fishbone diagrams (categories of causation), *25*, 52–53
    tree diagrams (chain of causes), 52–53
Centers for Medicare and Medicaid (CMS), 8
Chain of causes analysis. *See* Tree diagrams
Chart/file audits, 26
Checklists, 26
Chronic Care Model (CCM), 5–8, *6*
    clinical information systems, 7
    community, 7
    decision support, 7
    delivery system design, 7
    health systems, 6
    self-management support, 7
Chronic disease, 5
Clinic/institution specific measures, *14–15*
Continuous improvement cycle, 2
Continuous quality improvement (CQI)
    customer focus, 9–10, *9*
    definition of, 1
    emphasis on processes, 9
    use of objective data, 10
Correlation between variables. *See* Scatter diagrams
CQI and diabetes self-management education/support, 11–17
    audit items, 12–13
    benchmarking, 13, *13*
    CQI measures, *14–15*

HEDIS (Healthcare Effectiveness Data and
Information Set), 5
High-level flowcharts, 51
Histograms, 34–35, 54–55

**I**

Imai, Masaaki, 4
Improvement Tracker and Change Achievement
Success Indicator (IHI), 10
Improving Chronic Illness Care (ICIC), 6–7
Institute for Healthcare Improvement (IHI), 8–9,
10, 11
Institute of Medicine (IOM)
*Crossing the Quality Chasm*, 5
Internal/external customers, 9
International Organization for Standardization
(ISO), 3
Interviews, *26*
Ishikawa diagrams. *See* Fishbone diagrams

**J**

Japan, implementation of TQM, 3, 4
The Joint Commission, 5, 13, *14–15*
Just-in-Time (JIT), 4

**K**

Kaizen, 4

**L**

LEAN, 4
Look-up sample size chart, *28*

**M**

Matrix flowcharts. *See* Deployment/matrix
flowcharts
Measurable outcomes, 12
Motorola, 4

**N**

National Committee for Quality Assurance, 5
National Standards for Diabetes Management
Education and Support (NSDSME/S), 12, 16

**O**

Ordinal data, 25

Outcome measures vs. CQI measures, *23*
Outcomes continuum, *42*

**P**

Pareto charts, 29–30, *30*, 56
Pareto Principle, 29–30
Patient Protection and Affordable Care Act (ACA)
(2010), 4, 8–9
Patient safety, *13*
Patient-Centered Medical Home (PCMH), 8
Patient-defined goals, 12
Physician shortages, 9
Pie charts, 53–54
Plan-Do-Check-Act (PDCA), 2, *3*, 4
Plan-Do-Study-Act (PDSA), 2, 46–47, *47*
Plan implementation, 33–34
*The Principles of Scientific Management* (Taylor), 2
Privacy, 27
Problem identification, 22, *23*
Project leader, 20
Provider champion, 20

**Q**

QA storybooks/storyboards, 57
Quality assurance storytelling, 57
Quality control (QC), 2
Quality improvement process
evolution of, 2–4
QI process tools, *4*
Quality management (QM), 4

**R**

Ragged plateau histograms, 55
Research process. *See* CQI process and research
process
Robert Wood Johnson Foundation, 7, 10
Run charts, 28, 54

**S**

Sample size, 27–28, *28*
Scatter diagrams, 55–56
Scientific method, 2
Self-Care Behaviors Goal Sheet (AADE7™ System),
10, *17*, 21
Shewhart, Walter, 2–3